MAYDAY!

Captain John Winslow

CONTENTS

Published by Aerospace Publications Pty Ltd (ACN: 001 570 458) PO Box 1777, Fyshwick, ACT 2609, Australia.
Phone (02) 6280 0111, fax (02) 6280 0007, e-mail mail@ausaviation.com.au and website
www.ausaviation.com.au – publishers of monthly *Australian Aviation* magazine.
Production Manager: Gayla Wilson

ISBN 1-875671-56-0

Copyright © 2002 John Winslow and Aerospace Publications Pty Ltd
Proudly Printed in Australia by Pirie Printers Pty Ltd, 140 Gladstone St, Fyshwick, ACT 2609.
Distributed throughout Australia by Network Distribution Company, 54 Park St, Sydney, 2000. Fax (02) 9264 3278
Distributed in North America by Motorbooks International, 729 Prospect Ave, Osceola, Wisconsin, 54020, USA.
Fax (715) 294 4448. Distributed throughout Europe and the UK by Airlife Publishing Ltd, 101 Longden Rd,
Shrewsbury SY3 9EB, Shropshire, UK. Fax (743) 232944.

FRONT COVER ARTWORK BY PETE WEST

ACKNOWLEDGEMENTS

The production of this book would not have been possible on my own especially since reference material was not always easy to come by. I have to thank Macarthur Job, a well known Australian aviation and safety expert and author, for his ready and generous permission to use data from his previously published book *Air Disaster* and for his assistance with the 'detective work' of tracking down reference material. My long suffering wife fitted in her diligent proof reading between ironing, cooking and playing taxi driver to our children and gave many helpful and critical comments, she believes she deserves a large slice of the proceeds!

Captain John Williams, a friend of over 40 years, and now retired from his career in British Airways European Division, kindly read some of my initial efforts and greatly assisted in 'polishing' the stories to a readable level. To Captain Chris Wilson who put me in touch with the pilot of the Scimitar who bravely landed back on the aircraft carrier and Captain Robin Greenop who assisted in tracking down further reference material for that chapter and to Captain Peter Hessey and Alan Webber who kindly lent me that material, to them all many thanks. To the pilot who flew that aircraft, Mike Tristram (Royal Navy retired) I am deeply indebted for the time and trouble he took to provide data and then to comment on and correct the finished story and for his permission to reproduce his Queen's Commendation. His wingman Ben Bosworth also gave me his view of the episode and I thank him.

Thanks are due to Martin Emery, the First Officer on the ill fated 707 which landed at Istres. I relied heavily on his report to the press for the facts of this amazing incident which was kindly provided to me by aviation enthusiast Freddy Frost, an Air traffic Control Officer at Lasham Airfield in England

Captain Gordon Vette, a prominent New Zealand airline Captain, was instrumental in enabling me to write the account of the lost ferry pilot and his rescue before he finally ran out of fuel and had to ditch. Captain Vette himself played a major part in that rescue. I also acknowledge the valuable assistance of Stanley Stewart's account of this incident in his book *Emergency* published by Airlife. Eric Hoesing of the ever helpful Boeing Aircraft Company in Sydney provided valuable assistance with some technical details of the Boeing 707 aircraft which I had long ago forgotten.

Ken Lewis, the Manager Safety of the world's safest airline Qantas, was invaluable providing me with access to many accident and incident reports, thank you Ken. When those reports were unobtainable or missing, Russell Sibbison of Australia's Air Transport Safety Bureau kindly put me in touch with the US National Transportation Safety Board. Richard Kebabjian in the United States has a comprehensive website with details of many airline disasters and incidents, this was a great help in tracking material as was his personal intervention with details of the hard to find 1965 PanAm incident out of San Francisco – thank you Richard.

I am indebted to and acknowledge the assistance provided by the many reports in *Time* magazine and the *Washington Post* for the chronology and factual details of the extended hijack of TWA 847. Without their accurate reporting and their interviews with released passengers the full story of this incident could not have been told.

All official company reports of Captain Eric Moody's incredible encounter with volcanic ash have mysteriously disappeared off the face of the earth and without Betty Tootell's *All Four Engines Have Failed* (Andre Deutch Ltd in conjunction with Hutchinson (Australia) Pty Ltd, 1985) this epic story could not have been told. Her book provided many facts which were essential to writing an accurate account of the successful conclusion to a very ugly emergency. In am deeply indebted to Betty for permission to use her account as a basis for my rewrite of the incident. In the other British Airways incident, Captain My Captain, I initially relied heavily on the report by the UK Air Accident Investigation Board not being able to confirm the facts with BA authorities. Thanks to the British Airline Pilots' Association I was able to get in touch with Tim Lancaster and Alastair Atchison, the crew of the ill-fated BAC 111, their assistance was much appreciated and instrumental in correctly recording the facts of their frightening experience.

Joe Bracken, the Engineering and Accident Investigation representative of ALPA (the American Airline Pilots' Association) went to great trouble to provide me with otherwise unobtainable accident reports for reference and put me in touch with the son of the late Captain Testrake, hero of the hijack. This enabled me to confirm the accuracy of this chapter and provided some valuable personal details.

Not the least I must thank the publishers Aerospace Publications Pty Ltd and Jim Thorn in particular, who amazed me one morning by telling me that he thought the work worthy of publication.

INTRODUCTION

I was happy to be asked to introduce this book by Captain John Winslow so that I could express my admiration for the pilots and crew who feature in the various stories told. Written without any exaggeration or dramatisation they recount the factual details of control of the aircraft in almost impossible circumstances and the crew actions which averted what might have been fatal air crashes.

The intense and ongoing training of pilots is a great assurance to the travelling public and the selection procedures successfully choose those who can best handle the heavy responsibilities. The reader will certainly agree that there has always been something special about those who go about their business in aeroplanes both the cabin crew and pilots whom one Australian politician once called 'bus drivers'.

The book is one that can be picked up and put down since each chapter is an individual adventure story in itself. In fact it may be that the reader will find it so 'gripping' that one chapter at a time may be enough!

Throughout the book the author emphasises the continuing efforts of airline companies and aircraft manufacturers to improve aviation safety. Many of these safety improvements would not have been possible had it not been for the skills and bravery of the crews who brought the aircraft back and thus facilitated a thorough investigation of the problem. There is no doubt that all airline crews put safety before all else. I do hope you enjoy reading this book as much as I enjoyed reading the manuscript before publication.

Nancy Bird Walton,

Nancy-Bird Walton, A.O., O.B.E., Hon.D.Sc., Hon M.E.

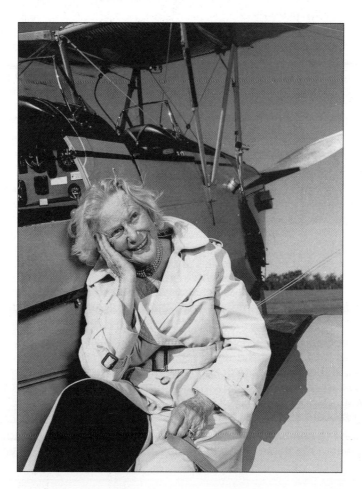

FOREWORD

There is no doubt that flying on a commercial airliner today is safer by far than the journey to the airport and it is becoming safer every day. Aircrew, both pilots and the cabin crew, are trained to an extremely high level and checked for health and proficiency on a regular basis. Their skills are constantly updated when new procedures or equipment come on line.

Each new generation of airliners incorporates the latest technology and, older airliners still in service are constantly upgraded. Aero engines which, in the early days of large piston engined airliners, when engines were turbocharged to the upper limits of their design capabilities, used to fail with monotonous regularity. With the advent of the basically simple jet engine they are becoming more and more reliable. Both the aircraft and engines are constantly checked and maintained meticulously. Why then do we from time to time learn of serious incidents or accidents affecting modern airliners?

No matter how much technology and training is applied, one cannot guard against the unknown. This is most vividly illustrated by the introduction of the first jet airliner, the de Havilland Comet. It flew into uncharted territory. Meticulously engineered and having gone through thorough and extensive test flying and certification checks, it nonetheless, suffered three major catastrophes with total loss of the aircraft and all those on board.

The Comet was the first pressurised large jet to operate regular scheduled services. It was later found that, flying at higher altitudes than any existing piston engined airliner, with increased pressure differentials between the cabin and the outside atmosphere, the repeated pressurisation and depressurisation of the hull as it climbed to cruise level and then descended to land at its destination, eventually caused a weakness of the hull which finally disintegrated with tragic results. This was new territory. Those problems were immediately rectified on the remaining aircraft and those subsequently built and the Comet went on to have an illustrious place in aviation history.

Modern generation aircraft are pressure tested for the planned number of 'cycles' (pressurisation and depressurisation) of the aircraft's life and then a healthy percentage on top of that. Wing bending capabilities are checked by testing a preproduction model to destruction. Engines are rigorously tested in many ways, not the least by firing semi defrosted chickens into the engine whilst it is running at full power to determine its capability to withstand major 'birdstrikes'. The engine manufacturers actually have a 'chicken gun' just for this purpose!

These days, computer design and many preconstruction test models can successfully eliminate post production problems for the airframe, operating systems and the engines, with the consequent and enormous increase in reliability and safety. There is unfortunately, as with all things mechanical, the smallest chance of a failure. Crews too are human and, as such are subject to human error although the crew selection and training procedures today are designed to minimise this possibility or, at very worst, contain a human error.

The safety factor built into airline operation today is that a specific failure cannot occur more than once in a hundred million hours. That is, if you take 75 years as an average lifespan, you would have to fly continuously for nearly 154 lifetimes before any specific failure occurred whilst you were on the aircraft! Safe enough for you?

Through the years as various aviation incidents have occurred, extensive enquires have been conducted with recommendations to prevent a repeat of the problem. The wreckage of an aircraft involved in a catastrophic crash is painstakingly reassembled, bit by bit in order to determine the exact cause and location of a failure. Inevitably, new mechanical problems come to light from time to time or unforeseeable natural phenomena manifest themselves. It is the pioneers who first experience these problems who have to resolve them with the skill and experience that they have. When they are able to successfully bring the aircraft back to land the investigators' task is greatly simplified. Many great safety advances have resulted from the evidence obtained from aircraft that have suffered a severe emergency, but have been brought 'home' enabling the investigating team to determine exactly what had happened.

Many current procedures for our big passenger jets have been derived as a result of these past unpleasant experiences and we are the safer for it. One good example which air passengers will observe on every flight is the security check to ensure that undesirable equipment is not being secretly carried on board. And then the lengthy delay whilst the baggage of a passenger who has not boarded is found and removed. A very sensible precaution since the missing passenger could well have secreted explosives on board and naturally, not want to travel on the aircraft.

Much has been done to combat terrorism and acts of mass murder. The reader should be assured that, when travelling with a reputable airline these days he is flying in a well maintained aircraft which has been serviced by highly trained engineers to the most exacting standards. The crew will have been trained in all aspects of safety and are very capable of dealing with any situation that may arise. Statistically you are safer in that aircraft than you are in your family car or even perhaps in your own home!

The following stories document some occasions when those incredible odds turned up and how the pilots and other crew battled against those odds to successfully (with one exception) bring the aircraft safely in to land. They are stories of incredible airmanship and courage. They vividly portray how modern airliners are built to the most exacting standards and, given the wrong circumstances, will still keep flying although severely crippled.

From each of these disasters have come changes to aircraft design, modification to aircraft systems and new procedures. These have all served to steadily increase airline safety to the high level it is today. The following chapters are testament to the courage and skill of the crews concerned and to the dedication and perseverance of the aircraft constructors and the airlines in the pursuit of increased safety.

I have avoided using inhouse technical aviation terms as much as possible but, inevitably, some technical details demand to be included. You may find your reading of the stories more enjoyable if you 'start at the back' with a glance through the glossary first.

Captain John Winslow
Sydney

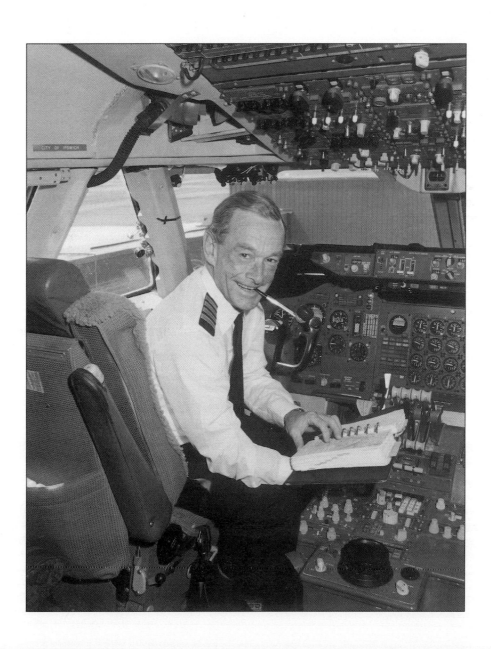

CHAPTER ONE

The Galunggung Incident

This incredible story of a crew's valiant and successful efforts to save a stricken Boeing 747 is given pride of place since it records what is recognised by many in the aviation industry as one of the greatest feats of airmanship and sheer guts in the history of commercial aviation.

That accolade is not only accorded to the pilots and engineer who were in the cockpit, but to the stewards and stewardesses who had no reason to believe they were going to survive but still kept their calm demeanour and went about their various tasks reassuring the passengers and preparing them and the cabin for what appeared to be an impending and catastrophic night ditching. All crew of passenger aircraft are very highly trained to deal with a wide variety of emergencies and problems but when there is no apparent reason for a problem and no procedure to deal with it, one can imagine the extreme concern and fear it must cause. The awards the crew received from many industry bodies are testimony to the courage and skill of the whole crew of Speedbird 9.

British Airways flight 009, callsign Speedbird 9, departed London Heathrow airport on June 23rd 1982 bound for Auckland via Bombay, Kuala Lumpur, Perth and Melbourne. The aircraft was a Boeing 747 registration G-BDXH. Although it lost a little time on its schedule the flight was perfectly normal to Kuala Lumpur where a routine crew change took place. The cockpit crew had brought the previous service in to Kuala Lumpur whilst the cabin crew had been positioned in from their last service to Jakarta. They now joined up to crew the Speedbird 9 to Perth.

It was a 'normal day at the office'. The crew departed their hotel in Jakarta and travelled to the airport. The cabin crew, under the direction of Cabin Service Officer Graham Skinner, boarded the aircraft and commenced to make the cabin ready for the arrival of the passengers and to receive and stow the catering for the ensuing flight. CSO Skinner assigned the crew their various positions and duties for the flight.

The flight engineer, Senior Engineer Officer Barry Townley-Freeman was also at the aircraft carrying out his preflight checks whilst Captain Eric Moody and Senior First Officer Roger Greaves were at flight planning checking the NOTAMS and weather and ordering the fuel they required for the flight after which they also proceeded to the aircraft to carry out their preflight cockpit checks and check the aircraft documentation. The passengers were boarded, the pilots received their clearance to depart for Perth and the aircraft made a normal departure, albeit still running a little behind schedule due to the late arrival of the flight into Kuala Lumpur.

The route along the airways to Perth passed close by the island state of Singapore, and then into Indonesian airspace just crossing the eastern coast of Sumatra, close to the Sunda Straits between Java and Sumatra and overhead Halim airport VOR. After crossing the densely populated island of Java, it took them in a southwesterly direction across the Indian Ocean to make their next landfall near Shark Bay in Western Australia.

Night had fallen and they had climbed to Flight Level 370. The weather in these tropical regions is usually very cloudy, often with substantial thunderstorms up to and above the cruising height of the jets, so a constant check of the weather radar was needed, as well as 'eyeballing' the telltale lightning flashes, to avoid undue turbulence. Unexpected entry into a thundercloud (cumulonimbus) can cause violent turbulence and injure both passengers and crew who are not securely strapped in.

In the 'two pilot' configuration which they were operating for this relatively short flight to Perth, it is normal procedure for each pilot and the engineer to take the occasional short time off to stretch their legs. Just after passing overhead the Halim VOR, Captain Moody elected to take a short break. He checked the weather radar to ensure that there was no adverse weather in the offing when it would be essential to have both pilots on duty. With no weather showing on the screen he duly handed over control to the First Officer and left the cockpit. Unfortunately the upstairs toilet was occupied so he proceeded to the lower deck.

Not long after the Captain had left the cockpit a series of unusual events began to unfold. The remaining crew noticed a St Elmo's Fire effect outside the windscreen. They had seen St Elmo's Fire often, but this was different. Little white sparks appeared to be flying at them giving the impression of flying through a snowstorm. St Elmo's Fire usually indicates that the aircraft is flying through cloud or in close vicinity of a thunderstorm.

In either case action was required. A further check of the weather radar did not indicate any weather ahead so the F/O switched on the landing lights and got the impression that they were indeed flying through thin upper cloud. As a precaution he put the seat belt sign on and the Flight Engineer switched on the engine anti-ice system. As an added precaution and to keep the Captain fully in the picture, the F/O requested one of the stewardesses to ask the Captain

Very soon after completing the engine shutdown drill for number 4 engine, number 2 engine surged and immediately flamed out. In quick succession this was followed by the failure of the last two operating engines.

to return to the flight deck. They were now about to cross the southern coast of Java.

In the passenger cabin, with the lights down low and just a few reading lights on, a thin film of smoke became evident swirling in the light beams much as would be expected if a few of the passengers were smoking cigarettes. The cabin air in the Jumbo completely changes every few minutes as outside air is drawn in, compressed, fed to the cabin and then vented out again through the 'outflow valves' which control the cabin pressure. Smoke from cigarettes will not linger long. On this occasion though the smoke continued to thicken and was evidently not normal and the cabin crew commenced a check of the cabin in their area to ensure a cigarette had not set fire to a seat or been discarded in the waste bins in the toilets, igniting used tissues and the like. Nothing was found, but, when they detected an acrid smell associated with the smoke, it was time to alert the CSO.

The Captain received the message to return to the flight deck and as he moved along the upper deck he also noticed the smoke, but it was not coming from smokers, it was seeping in through the many air conditioning vents along the upper cabin and when he opened the cockpit door he realised that the smoke was in the cockpit too.

He quickly got into his seat, strapped in and was immediately confronted by the amazing display of St Elmo's Fire which had now intensified and was unique in his vast experience. Before he could comment the F/O glanced out of his side window at the engines only to see yet another and even more amazing sight. The engine intakes were brilliantly illuminated by what seemed to be strong white light inside the engine. He could clearly see right inside the engine and a stroboscopic effect made it appear as if the giant first stage fan blades were rotating slowly backwards. Normally invisible with the high speed rotation, there were the blades individually visible. The leading edges of the wing were illuminated too by a diffuse white glow. It was the same on the Captain's side and the CSO who had come to the cockpit also saw this rare display, knew it wasn't normal and could presage trouble and possible turbulence. He left the flight deck immediately to prepare the cabin for what could be a rough ride to come.

The flight deck crew were now totally puzzled, there was nothing on the weather radar, there were no abnormal engine readings and nothing on the engineer's panel to indicate a malfunction which might be causing the smoke but the smoke was certainly coming from somewhere. It could be a developing air conditioning problem or an embryo electrical fire which had yet to manifest itself as a warning on the panel – it had that certain smell. Without the benefit of a warning light or unusual gauge reading there was no way to find the cause without a lengthy 'trouble shoot'.

Without a laid down procedure the crew were discussing what action should be taken when they got their first indication. A warning light flickered on the engineer's panel indicating a pneumatic problem. Before he could commence the standard procedure number four engine surged.

You do not need warning lights or instruments to detect a surge on a Boeing 747 engine. There is a distinct rumble and one can feel the momentary slight loss of power in the aircraft's movement. On the engine instrument panel up front and right in front of the pilots, a noticeable flicker in the engine speed and temperature was immediately followed by the engine flaming out – the engine was no longer providing any power.

"Confirm number four engine" called the Captain.

"Number four engine confirmed" replied the Flight Engineer.

"Number four thrust lever close. Number four start lever cutoff. Number four engine fire switch pull."

The Captain called the memory items for engine failure and the Engineer Officer, meticulously identifying each control from the four available, carried out the action confirming it to the Captain. They then completed the 'Loss of One Generator' procedure, ensuring power supply was fully available on the remaining three generators.

These procedures were routine and practised regularly in the simulator. It was not a great emergency. The aircraft could, in many circumstances, proceed to its destination on three engines at a slightly reduced altitude. However, this failure was different and very worrying. What had caused the flameout? The next action was to attempt to restart the engine.

Back in the cabin many passengers had seen the brilliant glow coming from the engines and the display of St Elmo's Fire along the leading edge of the wings. Coupled with the rapidly increasing density of the smoke in the cabin, some were convinced that the aircraft was on fire and, understandably, a slight element of panic started to set in. The cabin crew were well aware of the situation and set about securing the cabin for what might eventuate. To prevent further unease amongst the passengers they moved purposefully but quietly around the cabin completing their tasks and reassuring everyone.

The loss of number four engine and the fact that it would not restart immediately meant that, despite the application of maximum continuous power on the remaining three engines, the aircraft had to make a gentle descent to the three engine altitude where they could maintain level flight. Very soon after completing the engine shutdown drill for number 4 engine, number 2 engine surged and immediately flamed out. In quick succession this was followed by the failure of the last two operating engines.

All four engines had failed within the space of two minutes. They were without power and headed down toward mountainous terrain. Their electrical power would revert to a limited life battery, most of their instruments would fail and it would not be long before they lost cabin pressurisation. The situation was extremely grim and, in their experience, totally without precedent.

The First Officer put out a Mayday call to Jakarta informing them that they had lost all four engines and were descending. It was up to Jakarta to clear other aircraft who might be below them on the airway out of their descent path and to assist where possible. As is often the case in regions where the controllers' native language is not English and a non routine radio call is made, the controller had trouble grasping the dramatic content of the F/O's message and replied by enquiring whether Speedbird 9 had a problem!

Displaying remarkable restraint the F/O repeated the message only to have the Air Traffic Controller enquire whether it was number 4 engine that they had lost. All the time they were descending through altitudes at

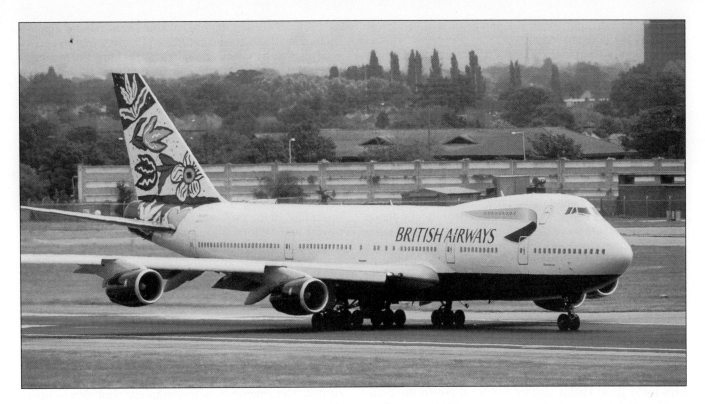

A British Airways Boeing 747-200. (Paul Merritt)

which other aircraft were possibly flying and who needed to be warned. Finally, with the assistance of a Garuda aircraft relaying the message, ground control became aware of the severity of the problem facing Speedbird 9.

Captain Moody was in an impossible situation. He was over high ground and could not descend below the safety height without risk of impact with the ground. The safety height was well over the altitude they would need to fly if the aircraft depressurised. He did not know if the engines would restart and was imminently going to lose much of his navigation and communication equipment with all the generators going offline with the engines failed yet, all the time, he needed to preserve precious height to give him time to get the engines restarted. A further problem was that the recommended height for engine starts was considerably lower than their present altitude although restarts are possible at higher altitudes. He had to decide to give the restarts a better chance or save his precious altitude.

A normal descent with the engines at idle will carry a 747 about 120 miles and takes just over 20 minutes. There would be a slight reduction in these figures with the engines totally failed and providing no thrust. That was all the time and distance Captain Moody had to somehow bring the stricken aircraft safely back to earth (or sea) and attempt a deadstick landing if the engines would not restart.

The Captain elected to turn back towards the main Jakarta Halim airport in anticipation that all would be well and they could land normally under power. He requested help from the radar controllers. At the current altitude and range from the airport they should have been clearly visible on radar but not only was there no trace on the radar screen of Speedbird 9, even the emergency code on their radar transponder was not showing. Radio transmission and reception was becoming ex-

tremely distorted and conversation with the controllers became increasingly more difficult.

As they continued attempts to restart the engines they had slowed the aircraft to the recommended speed for optimum engine relight capability. It was then they noticed there was a marked discrepancy between their airspeed indicated on the Captain's and F/O's airspeed indicators. The Captain decided to fly a speed averaging out the two airspeed readings to give them the best chance. It had no immediate affect but it revealed another problem that their pressure driven instruments were also now unreliable.

The inevitable loss of cabin pressure then hit them announced by the cabin warning horn indicating that the cabin altitude, normally around 5000 to 6000 feet had risen to over 10,000 feet. This called for the pilots and engineer to don their oxygen mask to ensure sufficient supply of oxygen and at worst, prevent them passing out. In the cabin the oxygen masks would soon fall from their ceiling stowages and the cabin crew would immediately take a seat and put on the nearest mask so that they too would remain useful to the operation.

The F/O pulled on his mask from the quick release stowage only to find that it was malfunctioning. Since the cabin altitude had only just reached 10,000 feet he still had some time before lack of oxygen would cause him to pass out but the Captain was concerned. He could not afford an incapacitated crewmember in this situation. He elected to increase the rate of descent of the aircraft to quickly reach a low altitude where oxygen would not be required but in doing so he was losing precious height and time and could not glide as far to possible safety.

If the engines could not be restarted he was facing a deadstick ditching in the sea at night, a feat never before performed and without any knowledge of the sea state. It was a difficult manoeuvre even with engine power and in daylight, at night, with no power, it would almost certainly result in a disaster.

The Senior Engineer Officer was working hard on the engineer's panel attempting to get the engines restarted and to analyse the reason for the failures. He covered all possible contingencies but there was no apparent reason and restarts were not successful. With the engines failed and the generators no longer supplying electricity, already the instruments and navigation equipment were failing; radios were extremely scratchy making communications with the ground almost impossible and, in the cabin, the lighting going on and off did nothing to reassure the passengers and cabin crew.

Nothing was going by the book. Theoretically many more instruments were operating than should have been with the power loss and some were behaving in a manner which had never been covered in simulator training.

The F/O managed to sort out the problem with his oxygen mask and Captain Moody was able to come back to a normal rate of descent and preserve precious altitude. However, they were now getting very close to the safety altitude, a height below which they could not descend due to the mountainous terrain below them. If they were not able to restart the engines the critical decision would have to be made and they would have to turn away from Halim airport and head out to the comparative safety over water giving them a little more time to continue the attempts to restart the engines.

Jakarta control, being unable to communicate with the crippled aircraft, now attempted to get another aircraft to relay messages from them but even this aircraft at cruise altitude could only just hear the frantic radio calls from Speedbird 9.

Trying to contact the Cabin Services Officer to inform him of the gravity of the situation and to order the cabin prepared for a ditching, Captain Moody found that the cabin service interphone was not functioning. He also needed to inform the passengers of what was happening but even the Public Address System was malfunctioning and his message only partly got through. He was able though to order the CSO to the flightdeck.

Radio communications with Jakarta were still almost impossible as the static on the radio made it very hard to hear or be heard. The F/O finally got through and requested the aircraft's position on radar. Jakarta could not see the aircraft on its screen and requested their position from the Halim VOR but this was not being received so F/O Greaves gave them a distance and bearing from the one remaining INS and were told by Jakarta not to descend below 12000 feet, the minimum safe height in this mountainous area – easier said than done!

As they got ever closer to the safety height they frantically continued the relight attempts and at last number 4 engine responded. Whilst the four engined 747 can fly on one engine at low weights and at low altitude, one engine would not be enough to maintain an altitude above the safety height, but it was a start. It also gave them limited electrical power as that engine's generator came back on line.

Their efforts were rewarded when a short while later number 3 engine restarted. That meant they would be able to stay above safety height but the question was what damage had the engines suffered and would they stay operational? It would not be prudent to proceed over the mountain chain and have them fail again.

Captain Moody minimised the strain on the engines by leaving them at one setting and abandoned his previous plan to turn out to sea for a ditching. At last after more restart attempts the remaining two engines started and they were able to request a climb to a higher level to give them a bigger safety margin should further trouble eventuate. They climbed to FL 150, (15,000 feet) and were able to receive the Halim VOR which told them they were 108 miles away to the south-southeast.

Suddenly it was all returning to normal; Jakarta then picked them up on radar which took a big load off the crew since they could now be navigated by the ground controllers using the radar. With all four engines now operating all the previous problems of reduced electrical power and lack of pressurisation had gone away. They now only needed to nurse the aircraft to a landing at Halim and let the ground engineers take over problem solving the failures.

As they neared their new altitude though, the St Elmo's fire effects which had dissipated, returned. It was now obvious that there was a connection with these phenomena and the engine failures so the Captain immediately started down again to near to, but above, the safety height. Before he could make a reduction in the altitude number 2 engine commenced a series of violent surges. The engine was immediately shut down again; three engines working normally were enough for their needs and they did not need one rogue engine disrupting their attention.

Captain Moody was now fairly confident that everything was under control and passed the good news to the passengers and crew on the PA, announcing that they expected to be landing at Jakarta shortly. He was well aware that they were all very shaken and needed any reassurance he could afford them. They passed over the mountain range and were cleared lower for their approach to land. Not wishing to tempt fate the Captain tried to keep the engine thrust setting constant and varied height by using the speedbrake effecting a steady and gentle descent towards Halim airport.

A check on the weather (they were going to Halim in any event) indicated that at least the weather had been kind to them, it was a nice night and calm. To ease the strain the captain, who had been hand flying for some time now, engaged the autopilot but it would not lock in. Happily the second autopilot functioned and he was able to take some load off himself to prepare for the landing.

They were transferred to Jakarta approach control who cleared them to continue their approach and asked if they required assistance on arrival. Not knowing what had caused all their problems they requested that the fire services be prepared for their landing.

It soon became apparent that their prudent and gentle treatment of the engines had left them a little high for a straight in approach so a turn was requested to lose height for landing and they made a 'procedure turn' over an approach radio beacon. They then discovered that the glidepath component of the instrument landing system was out of order for their arrival and that they would have to judge their descent to land visually. Not a hard task and one practised frequently in the simulator but not really needed at the end of a gruelling emergency.

They flew ever closer to the airport when the F/O noticed that the airport lights were apparently affected by mist, not reported on the weather report they had

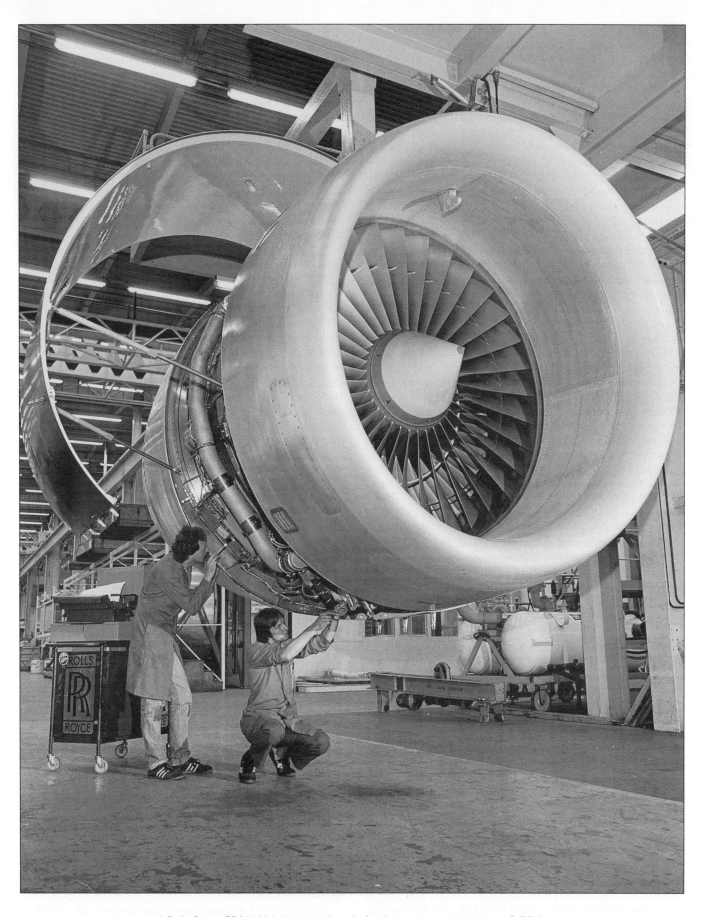

A Rolls-Royce RB211 high bypass ratio turbofan the same as used to power G-BDXH.

earlier received. In case it was moisture on the outer windscreen they operated the windscreen wipers and washers with no change to the view of the airport. It rapidly became clear that the outer windscreen had suffered considerable damage and this was the cause of their lack of clear forward vision.

By getting the airfield lighting turned up to full brilliance and with the Captain squinting through the extreme edge of his forward windscreen panel which was less severely affected, they made their approach. F/O Greaves kept the distance measuring equipment switched on on his side so that he could provide a cross check on the approach which is almost exactly 300 feet per mile out. When the landing lights were switched on for the landing there was no result, obviously they had suffered in the same way as the windscreen but the VASIS did come into view. They would have been a great help in making a safe landing. They completed the approach operating as they had been trained to do with the F/O cross checking and assisting the Captain and the engineer officer backing them both up.

They touched down and the roar of the reverse thrust told the passengers that they were finally safely back on terra firma. Cheers and clapping broke out in the cabin. They taxied in to the parking bay with extreme care and difficulty, the vision through the windscreen was so poor it made safe manoeuvring difficult even on the ground. A 'follow me' vehicle was requested but the ramp floodlighting, diffused through the windscreen made it impossible to move safely to their parking position so the final few yards were made under tow and they came to a stop almost exactly one hour after the terror had begun. They had arrived!

As they disembarked from the aircraft the extent of the damage became evident. The wings and engine pods had been 'sandblasted' to the bare metal, the windscreen and landing light covers were opaque. There was very evident severe damage to the engines themselves and all around there was the presence of a fine, talcum like grey dust. It all became clear, they had unwittingly flown into a cloud of volcanic ash.

The Indonesian island of Sumatra has a chain of high ground running along its southern side. Most of the mountains are volcanic and, by the definition of vulcanologists, most are active. It was at the western end of Java in August 1883 that the volcanic island of Krakatoa exploded sending out a 130 metre high tidal wave that killed over 36,000 people. The volcanic dust remained in the atmosphere for over a year. Small rocky pinnacles in the Sunda Strait are the only remains of the island today. At the eastern end of Java just a few years earlier in 1815 Mount Tambora on the island of Lombok had exploded throwing massive amounts of debris and dust into the sky. The eruption had six million times the energy of an atomic bomb. It took several months until it cleared or settled back to earth.

Mount Galunggung, the villain of this story, is a small mountain by volcanic standards, just 2168 metres high, and lies around 255 kilometres to the east south east of Jakarta. In the early 1800's there were two significant eruptions causing many deaths and much destruction then, after another less severe eruption in 1890, there

was a long period of quiescence with only minor rumblings until early April 1982 when the distinct rumblings and tremors presaging an eruption began. For several days minor eruptions occurred and lava flows threatened surrounding villages which were evacuated. The whole countryside became covered in ash. On June 24th increasingly violent eruptions commenced. Huge boulders were thrown from the crater and, with a final 'tour de force' the mountain exploded sending cloud of ash and particles up into the stratosphere where it drifted on the upper winds into the airway along which Speedbird 9 was flying to Perth.

The nature of volcanic ash is rather like fine talcum powder. It gets into every nook and cranny and simply asphyxiates a jet engine. In the hot part of the engine it will bake onto the turbine blades unbalancing them and further disrupting the engine's normal operations. Volcanic ash, however, does not show up on an aircraft's weather radar which is calibrated precisely to pick up only water droplets.

The successful recovery from this severe emergency undoubtedly constitutes one of the finest feat of airmanship on record and the conduct of the cabin crew in every way complemented the work in hand in the cockpit. All the crew received recognition and awards for their skills including Captain Moody's Queen's Commendation for Valuable Service in the Air, and further awards by The British Airline Pilots' Association and the Guild Of Air Pilots & Navigators, Lloyds of London, who insured the aircraft and, of course, British Airways. The whole crew was honoured by a dinner at the Guildhall in London hosted by Lloyds of London

As a result of this incident, airlines, in conjunction with the aircraft manufacturers developed special procedures to deal with encountering a volcanic ash cloud but, more importantly, all volcanos world wide which could affect air routes are now monitored by satellite on a continuous basis and alerts are provided to the aviation authorities whenever an eruption presents any possibility of a repeat of this near disaster. These alerts are rapidly passed on to airlines and the crews and alternate routes to avoid trouble are planned or, in extreme cases, the flight postponed.

THE AIRCRAFT AND CREW

British Airways Flight BA009 departed London Heathrow on June 23rd 1982. The aircraft was Boeing 747 registration G-BDXH named City of Edinburgh. The flight was scheduled to operate from London to Bombay flying on to Kuala Lumpur, Perth, Melbourne and Auckland.

The cabin crew and technical aircrew joined up in Kuala Lumpur The 13 cabin crew were headed by Cabin Service Officer Graham Skinner, deadheaded in from Jakarta. The rest of the cabin crew were Purser Sarah de Lane Lea, Fiona Wright, Geoffrey Bell, Araf Chohan, Purser Richard Abrey, Stewardesses Lorraine Stewart, Claire Wickett, Susan Glennie and Stewards Bernard Martin, Roger MacNichol, Nicholas Grey and Stephen Johns.

The technical aircrew were Captain Eric Moody, Senior F/O Roger Greaves and SEO Barry Townley-Freeman.

CHAPTER TWO

Martin Baker Let Down

I include this personal account since it illustrates how often an aircraft accident is built up from a series of minor occurrences and how, in exceptional circumstances, the million to one odds of the accident happening at all are sometimes offset by a million to one escape from a futureless conclusion.

It is also a fine example that these things always seem to happen at exactly the wrong time and place! It also gave me personal experience of two strange phenomena which humans experience, which I can confirm do happen and are quite amazing.

HMS *Bulwark*, one of the Royal Navy's light fleet carriers, was to carry out an 'open day' cruise off the coast of Aden, a bit of what was known in the Navy as 'flag waving'. Invited on board for the day to watch flying operations first hand were senior representatives of the Royal Air Force, the Army, local dignitaries and the press.

No 801 Seahawk day fighter squadron and 891 squadron operating the Sea Venom night fighter aircraft were to be launched and carry out various demonstrations and fly-pasts. The launch and subsequent land on would be excitement enough for our visitors since they are both spectacular to watch.

The weather was fine and, as usual off Aden, very hot. The sea was choppy with about two metre waves but nothing to cause undue movement of the carrier and upset our guests. Captain Percy Gick, commanding officer, turned the carrier into wind and the ship's speed was increased to give the required windspeed over the deck for aircraft launch. Signal flag 'foxtrot' was hoisted indicating that flying operations were now in operation.

The Seahawks of 801 squadron were ranged on the deck, engines running ready for the launch, behind them the Sea Venoms of 891 squadron, ready to follow in short order. We were looking for a slick launch to impress our visitors, however, it is always an important consideration in any event since the carrier in wartime is very vulnerable keeping one course for any length of time during a launch and it is extremely important to get all aircraft off in the minimum amount of time.

My commanding officer's aircraft was loaded onto the port catapult, as I was loaded onto the starboard catapult as his number two. The Flight Deck Officer gave the signal for full power and having got the thumbs up from the CO, lowered his flag to order the launch. With an enormous kick, even from the new steam catapults, the CO's aircraft took to the air and I immediately received the signal to apply full power. All was well, instruments all checked out and I indicated ready for launch.

The Flight Deck Officer lowered his flag and I was off but this launch was far from normal! There was a large explosion, the cockpit filled with smoke and the aircraft vibrated so badly I could not read the instruments. I was partly stunned, I later learnt that it was because my head had struck the top of the cockpit with some force, and my first recollections were that the sea was coming up to meet me and that the aircraft was not going to accelerate away.

It is said that time apparently slows in an emergency. It certainly did for me that day; it seemed to come to a complete standstill. There was actually a little over seven seconds from the moment of launch until the aircraft hit the sea yet I had more than enough time to think out the problem and the pros and cons of any action, or lack of action that I might take. I was sitting immediately in front of a jet engine revolving at an extremely high speed and very hot and about to land in the relatively cool seawater.

My first thought was that the engine could explode so I took all power off and, realising that ditching was imminent and that I was too low to eject, I reached for the canopy jettison handle. That was my last recollection prior to coming round underwater.

Needless to say back on deck, the air display launch was immediately cancelled and our visitors were treated to a real life rescue of a downed pilot. But what had happened and how did it happen? It was some time later before all the circumstances were revealed.

> *Realising that ditching was imminent and that I was too low to eject, I reached for the canopy jettison handle. That was my last recollection prior to coming round underwater.*

A movie film is taken of every aircraft launch and landing so there is a visual record should an accident occur. It revealed that, immediately the launch commenced a projectile had fired upwards through my canopy deploying a small parachute which had immediately opened fully and decelerated the aircraft causing it to head downwards. It was known that this was the ejection seat stabilising parachute which deploys on a normal ejection preventing the seat from tumbling, injuring the pilot and ensuring normal operation of the pilot's personal parachute.

This 'chute operates on the first upwards movement of the seat on a normal ejection. The movement of the seat triggers a charge that fires a steel rod which in turn pulls the stabilisation 'chute out of its stowage. It was this steel rod which had first pieced my aircraft canopy. Unfortunately, the initial movement of the seat also triggers a barostat which releases the possibly unconscious pilot from the seat if the ejection takes place below 10,000 feet, the object being to descend him quickly still in the ejection seat from higher altitudes which are not

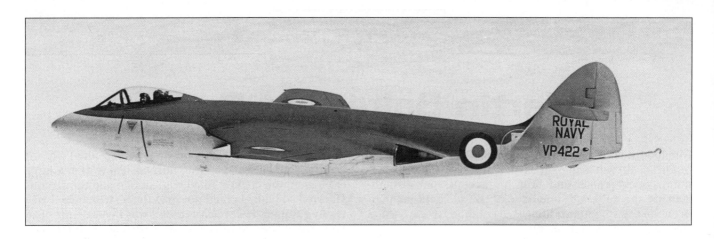

A Hawker Seahawk identical to that flown by the author. (BAe)

environmentally friendly to the human frame! Being at very low altitude, the seat movement had also released my seat harness immediately before a ditching at something in excess of 140mph!

The question then arose as to what had permitted the ejection seat to move at all when it is tightly secured to the aircraft structure by two locks until the explosive charge is operated by the pilot pulling 'the blind' to eject. Obviously one or more of the locks had failed.

Investigations determined that the lower of the two locking latches had released allowing movement of the seat. This latch had to be installed by hand but this had to be done 'blind' since it was situated beneath the rear of the seat when it was installed in the aircraft. Worse still, it could be put in upside down and had no safeguards such as a channel or lug on the lock to prevent incorrect insertion.

Murphy had struck and the bottom-locking latch on my aircraft had been installed upside down with catastrophic results – human error and an understandable one at that but, more pertinently, a manufacturing oversight and an accident waiting to happen.

So how am I now writing this account of my own serious aircraft accident?

The million to one odds *in my favour* came up at the exact second I needed them. A crippled aircraft, ditching in a rough sea (for any swimmer) at a high speed and right in front of a 27,000 ton aircraft carrier bearing down at 25 knots! Not a good scenario to start with but then remember, my seat harness had released!

Regretfully, the photographer had ceased filming just after my launch not noticing through his viewfinder that he was about to get some very interesting footage. Had he kept filming it would have shown the canopy flying free as I jettisoned it a split second before the aircraft hit the water and, as the canopy left the aircraft, so did I. The upward movement of the malfunctioning ejection seat had been arrested by the remains of the shattered canopy. It was only when I jettisoned the canopy before impact that the seat, with me still seated in it, was pulled clear of the stricken aircraft by the very drogue 'chute which had caused the ditching in the first place.

It wasn't quite over yet. Due to concussion I was unaware that I had had both eyelids nearly torn off in the impact with the sea and had lost all sight due to swelling, my lifesaving Mae West was ripped open and useless, my personal parachute had broken free from its pack and I

was severely tangled in the parachute shroud lines and the impact had ripped off my two calf length laced up flying boots.

I knew that I was underwater and instinctively swam upwards. The rescue helicopter was overhead, a crewman in the water beside me trying to get me into the lifting harness but he too became tangled in the parachute shroud lines and had to be rescued. At least I was partially in the lifting strop and could hang on to the lifting wire and take a rest. I breathed in as each wave trough passed and held my breath whilst the waves passed over me. It was just a matter of time before I was rescued I thought.

Suddenly the lifting wire went slack and I fell back into the sea. I later discovered that the helicopter was about to be rammed by the carrier and had to release the line to get out of the way. They could not lift me back on board anyway since, being tangled in the main parachute lines; they would have had to lift a huge parachute full of seawater as well as myself. A weight far beyond the capabilities of the of the S-55 Whirlwind rescue helicopter.

Eyewitnesses say that the ship passed about ten feet away from me aided by the violent emergency manoeuvre the Captain had initiated on seeing an aircraft imminently ditching. I was now well aware that I was drowning and it was actually quite pleasant. There was a warm soft feeling about it and if there had been an orchestra handy, violins would have been playing relaxing music! Despite the pleasant feelings I preferred not to die by drowning.

I heard voices nearby, the lifeboat, launched the instant it became obvious an aircraft was ditching to back up the helicopter, had reached me. I vividly remember shouting at the top of my voice "For Christ's sake get me out of here" only to realise that not a sound had come from my mouth I was so exhausted and near to death.

I felt strong hands grasp me under the armpits and haul me over the boat's gunwale where I rested for a few moments while a seaman cut free the many shroud lines entangling me. I was then brought into the boat and laid in the scuppers for the ride back to the ship. The lifeboat was shackled onto the davits, raised and brought in board. I was hustled away on a stretcher, down the bomb lift to the sick bay.

The Surgeon Commander examined me. He did not mention that both my eyelids were hanging off nearly

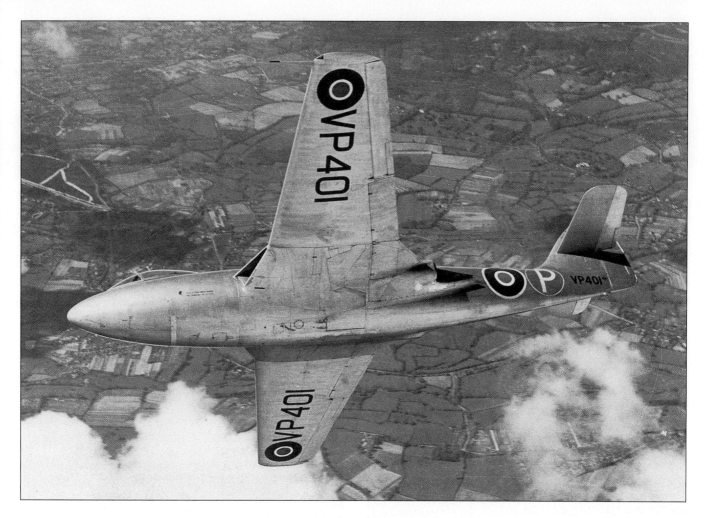

The Seahawk was very popular with its pilots, many describing it as the nicest aircraft they had ever flown. This is the prototype wearing RAF colours prior to the type becoming a naval fighter. (BAe)

severed but said I had a few minor scratches and one other injury which puzzled him. He could not understand why I had a fresh, third degree burn on my buttock. It turned out that my rescuers had laid me on the lifeboat's exhaust pipe for the run back to the ship. I hadn't felt a thing!

By curious quirk of fate, at the RAF hospital at Steamer Point, there was a visiting RAF plastic surgeon who had come out from the UK to rebuild the face of an airman who had had a rocket explode whilst it was being loaded onto an aircraft. He was able to operate on my eyelids and restore me to normality.

Had I not jettisoned the canopy at the exact moment that I did I would have still been in the aircraft as it hit the sea and would have been thrown violently against the gunsight and forward instrument panel and undoubtedly killed. It was 9.01am on the 18th of August 1958 – I remember it well!

I resumed flying duties after my recovery and rejoined the same squadron, still under the command of the same CO. We embarked on board HMS *Centaur* for another operational cruise.

We were conducting a routine launch almost exactly one year after my accident when I was coincidentally again number two to the CO. He launched off the port catapult and through his canopy came the dreaded drogue chute bullet followed by the chute itself which deployed behind his aircraft. It was a carbon copy of my

accident. The CO however escaped from this situation in a very different way. He had been an instructor at The Empire Test Pilots' School at Farnborough, had been involved in the development and testing of many prototype aircraft and was a highly skilled and much decorated pilot.

Knowing immediately what had occurred (he had handled the investigation and report into my accident a year earlier) and knowing that he now had no seat harness, he placed his feet on the gunsight arch, the strongest part of the structure, and flew the aircraft into the sea looking between his feet. The aircraft immediately started to sink, water filled the cockpit and light began to fade as the aircraft went down. The ejection seat was now useless, even for an underwater ejection. He tried to push the remains of the canopy off to make his escape but it wouldn't budge.

He finally turned upside down in the cockpit and kicked it free with his feet, escaped from the cockpit and swam to the surface. On deck we saw him break the surface and give a vigorous wave to indicate his position and that he would like a lift but he immediately vanished below the surface again. He later told us that his personal parachute rigging lines had tangled round his neck the other end being snagged on the sinking aircraft. He freed himself and once more came to the surface to be rescued by the helicopter. Within five minutes of his accident he was into a stiff gin in the wardroom!

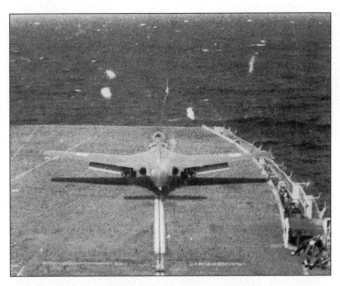 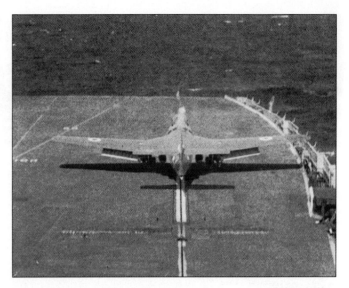

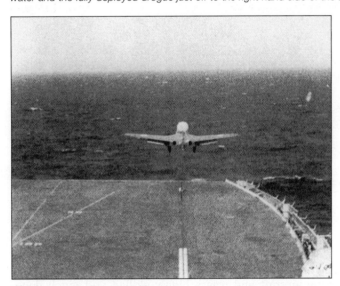 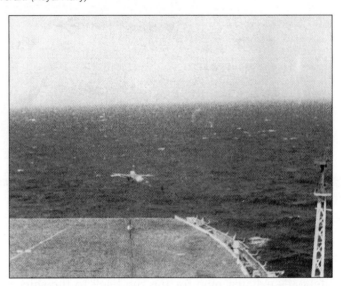

The series of events that almost cost a life. Pic 1 depicts the ejection seat commencing its firing procedure with the cable and drogue deployment bullet seen firing skywards from aft of the canopy area. Pic 2 depicts the emergence and initial inflation of the drogue chute. Pic 3 clearly shows the inflated drogue chute heading back towards the tailplane as the aircraft leaves the carrier while the final pic shows the aircraft about to impact the water and the fully deployed drogue just off to the right hand side of the aircraft. (Royal Navy)

When he had had a medical check up and was found to be undamaged, we invited him to the hangar deck to show us how he had ditched and turned upside down to kick the canopy free. Being something over six-foot tall it came as no surprise to us that he could achieve neither manoeuvre in the cold light of day. It is quite amazing what adrenaline can do when push comes to shove.

Quite understandably the CO initiated enquiries as to what had happened to the recommendations that we forwarded to Admiralty after my accident which included a lug on the bottom-locking latch to prevent it being inserted upside down. The recommendations were traced to the overflowing 'in tray' of a desk bound Admiralty clerk still not actioned after a year's lapse of time.

I had unwittingly flown the aircraft on its last flight before this launch. Part of the test flight I was to perform was an inverted flight test which checks out the functioning of the engine oil system in negative G conditions. I was unable to carry out this part of the test flight schedule and made a note on the test card and informed our Engineer Officer that it would have to be carried out on the next flight. Had I inverted the aircraft the seat would have fallen from the aircraft in

inverted flight and I would have suddenly found myself descending by parachute wondering where the aircraft had gone as had happened to quite a number of pilots in the past. I have never been so grateful for a hangover in all my life!

The development of the ejection seat by the Martin Baker company has been instrumental in saving the lives of thousands of military pilots flying jet aircraft. Without the seat pilots could not have successfully escaped from jet aircraft at high speed or great altitudes nor at the incredibly low levels at which emergencies sometimes occurred, even ground level with the latest seats.

The normal method of returning to earth in a military aircraft under radar or radio control is called a letdown. Consequently escape from a stricken aircraft using the ejection seat, with the subsequent descent by parachute, has become known in the trade as a 'Martin Baker Letdown'.

Like all machinery though, the seat has to be properly maintained and installed and this chapter is no reflection whatsoever on the wonderful device that Martin Baker invented which is highly valued by all military pilots around the world.

CHAPTER THREE

Beyond the Limits

The year was 1958, Captain Gordon Thain of British European Airways was the captain of an Airspeed Ambassador which failed to get airborne while attempting a takeoff in snow at Munich Airport.

In the subsequent crash a large number of the Manchester United UK soccer team perished or were severely injured along with other passengers. He had done everything right, the aircraft had simply not got airborne. For years Captain Thain fought to clear his name before it was finally realised that it was the retardation effects of the snow on the runway at Munich that had so slowed the aircraft that it did not reach flying speed. At that time no provision was made for such an eventuality and little was known about take-off in snow or slush. Happily he was finally cleared of culpability but his career had been ruined.

These days the thorough and all-embracing investigations that take place more often than not prevent such injustices, but it has to be admitted that pilots, being human, do make errors. The crew concept and rigorous training eliminate most of these but a new training development has also been introduced to eliminate situations where one pilot's mistake may go unchallenged by the other crewmembers; it is called Crew Resource Management.

The most junior pilot is directed to challenge the Captain if he or she is not fully satisfied that a decision or manoeuvre is totally safe and Captains are instructed to listen to advice from all their crewmembers regardless of experience or seniority. It was not always so!

The following incident starts with some undoubtedly poor airmanship on the part of some of the crew, but their subsequent efforts did save the aircraft and passengers aided and abetted by the incredible strength of the design of the Boeing 747SP aircraft in which they were fortunate enough to be flying that day.

The Boeing 747SP is a variant of the standard 747. Designed for longer range and low passenger density routes, the fuselage was shortened by some 14 metres and, due to the shorter moment arm reducing control effectiveness, the tailplane was enlarged. It carried a fraction more fuel than the standard aircraft and had other minor differences.

The consequence of all this was that it could reach much higher cruising levels at the beginning of the flight and had a greater range than the standard aircraft. The

Pointing straight towards earth, the sleek airframe of the 747SP allowed the airspeed to increase rapidly until they exceeded their limiting speed. Recovery from this unaccustomed attitude on instruments alone was hard enough but with their excessive speed, it would be very easy to overstress the already taxed airframe and that would mean only one thing – midair disintegration.

SP was used by Pan American World Airways to achieve the first Los Angeles to Sydney direct flights which could take up to 14 hours and longer.

China Air flight 006 was operating from Taipei across the Pacific to Los Angeles on the 29th of March 1985, a day the 274 passengers and crew would not forget. The 11 hour plus flight was just what this aircraft had been designed for but, to ensure that all crew remained rested, vigilant and alert, the normal three man crew of Captain Min-Yuan Ho, First Officer Ju Yu Chang and Flight Engineer Kuo-Pin Wei was supplemented by an extra Captain and Flight Engineer, Chien-Wan Liao and Shih Lung Su. The crew then took turns in the crew sleeping accommodation provided behind the cockpit area.

All the crew were highly qualified and, since the aircraft had been leased by China Air and still flew under an American registration, all the crew were required to hold US licences which they did.

The flight had proceeded quite normally for just under 10 hours and, as the fuel was used had progressively climbed to higher and more economic cruising levels. They had reached FL 410 (41,000 feet), which was well under the maximum permitted cruise altitude of 45,000 feet, and were flying 'in the clear' above a cloud layer. They were on the airway system around 300 nautical miles to the northwest of San Francisco just over an hour from top of descent when they began to encounter mild turbulence.

Cruising at Mach .85, the autopilot was controlling the aircraft under their watchful eyes but, at these higher altitudes, the autopilot was not handling the slight turbulence well, The thrust levers were 'hunting' as the computers tried to maintain the correct speed which was now varying between M.84 and M.88. As the airspeed once again started to decrease the autopilot computer programmed the throttles (thrust levers in aircraft parlance) to increase power. The three left hand engines all started to 'spool up' (accelerate) but despite the number four thrust lever moving forward, the engine power did not change.

The Flight Engineer, watched by the Captain, gently moved the number four thrust lever forwards and backwards but to no avail. The engine remained at the reduced power setting and, with insufficient power, the airspeed started to decrease. With the speed still decreasing they needed to take remedial action, either to

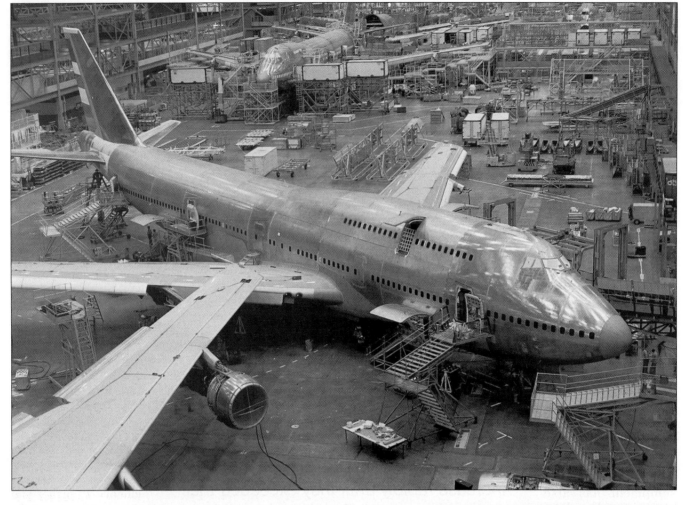

A Boeing 747, this one an extended upper deck -300 model, on the company's Everett production line outside Seattle. Always considered an ultra strong and very safe design, the 747 certainly proved its strength with what occurred via the China Airlines incident. (Boeing)

get the engine operating normally or to commence a descent to an altitude where they could maintain height on three engines.

By this time, due to other indications on the F/E's panel he became convinced that the engine had actually flamed out and the Captain ordered the engine shut down procedure and told the F/O to request a descent.

By now the autopilot, trying to correct the asymmetric thrust and the ever slowing airspeed, had applied the input to keep the aircraft level and the control wheel was deflected well to the left. The F/O, hearing the F/E tell the Captain that number four had flamed out, told the supernumerary F/E to come forward to assist. He saw that the speed was still decreasing and getting uncomfortably low and alerted the Captain and then called Oakland control and requested the descent. They did not hear Oakland reply a minute later with their clearance to descend, they were now concentrating hard on containing the situation.

The Captain, realising that they could not continue to maintain altitude with the reducing airspeed, adjusted the autopilot controls to commence a descent regardless whilst maintaining their correct track. By now the control wheel was deflected hard over as the computers struggled to prevent the aircraft rolling. Despite the entry into a descent the airspeed continued to fall.

The situation was now becoming dangerous and the Captain decided to disconnect the autopilot and to fly the aircraft manually into the much needed descent. The aircraft was already banked slightly to the right. When the autopilot was disconnected the flying control deflections from the autopilot's efforts were still in place. Before the Captain could make a correction the aircraft started to yaw and roll rapidly to the right causing the F/O to further alert the Captain.

The Captain was now concentrating hard on his attitude indicator, the so-called artificial horizon, watching carefully for the sign that his control inputs were again levelling the aircraft when the horizon suddenly went crazy, rolling rapidly and indicating a very steep descent. He glanced across to the F/O's instrument and to the third attitude indicator, they were the same and there were no failure flags.

At this moment they entered the cloud layer. In a few seconds they had rolled almost onto their back and entered a vertical dive – they were in a catastrophic jet upset. Fortunately the Captain had put the seat belt sign on earlier when they had encountered the turbulence and most passengers and crew were seated and strapped in.

Not so lucky the supernumerary Captain. He had woken up when the second F/E had been requested to come to the flightdeck. He had heard that they had lost an engine and decided to also go up to help. As he left the crew bunk he was thrown to the floor and pinned there. That was where he remained for the next few minutes totally unable to move his slight frame now

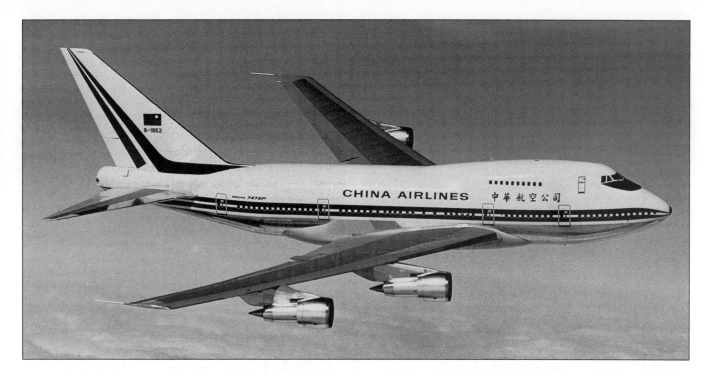

A China Airlines 747SP identical to the one portrayed in this chapter. (Boeing)

weighing several times its normal weight as huge G forces were experienced.

Pointing straight towards earth, the sleek airframe of the 747SP allowed the airspeed to increase rapidly until they exceeded their limiting speed. Recovery from this unaccustomed attitude on instruments alone was hard enough but with their excessive speed, it would be very easy to overstress the already taxed airframe and that would mean only one thing – midair disintegration.

It was vital that the wings were levelled before any attempt was made to recover from the dive, airlines are simply not built for high G rolling manoeuvres. All this time the speed was still increasing and they were diving towards the sea at a rate never considered by Boeing's designers.

The F/E believed that the other three engines had flamed out and was reporting this to the Captain at the very moment that they had lost control. Now he saw further instrument indications which confirmed his earlier report. Well aware that they would need the engines as soon as they regained level flight he set about restarting them. He checked for throttle response, there was none. He switched on the secondary ignition switches with no result but as he went to carry out further actions the Captain pulled back on the control column making further attempts to pull out of the dive. The F/E found himself pinioned by the G force. He could not lift his arms and his head was forced down against the central control pedestal, which was between the two pilots' seats.

The Captain was having great difficulty making sense of the instruments which were not designed to cope with the extreme attitudes they were experiencing. Now in cloud, they were his only attitude reference.

Finally he achieved some semblance of level flight and the attitude indicator started to make sense. He pulled back hard on the control column but as he continued to attempt recovery from a dive the rapidly deceasing airspeed told him that he had overshot level flight and was now climbing far too fast. The airspeed

decreased to well below the stall speed and he pushed hard forward on the controls experiencing negative G and the weightless feeling that accompanies it.

In the cabin the terrified passengers and crew were left wondering what had happened and what their fate would be. There had been no time for announcements, indeed it would have been impossible to reach out and pick up the microphone from its stowage. As the aircraft pulled out of a dive, they were pressed down in their seats by the massive G forces only a few moments later to find themselves almost weightless and their bodies straining against the seat belts as the aircraft nosed over only to repeat the cycle as the struggle to recover control continued. The constantly changing sound of the slipstream and the creaking strains of the structure further added to their alarm.

The Captain's struggles, watched by his more than anxious fellow crewmembers, continued. They were all aware that all the aircraft limitations of speed and G forces had been exceeded and wondered how long it would be before the terrible abuse would take its toll.

The incredible attitudes they had encountered all the while in cloud had added little to the success of the Captain's efforts. Spatial disorientation had now undoubtedly set in, the fluids in the inner ear tell you one thing, the instruments another. It is almost impossible to overcome the senses and believe the instruments after such a ride. It's like the party game of spinning someone blindfold, inevitably they will fall over, they need the visual reference to stay on their feet. Coupled with the lingering doubts about the reliability of his instruments, it became virtually impossible to effect a recovery while they were still in cloud.

Finally, at about 10,000 feet the aircraft flew into clear sky. Now, with a visual horizon to help, the Captain was able to rapidly get the aircraft levelled off. In the space of just over four minutes they had dived more than 30,000 feet and for some of that four minutes they had been going *up* in the overshoots they had experienced pulling out of the dives. The normal descent rate of a 747

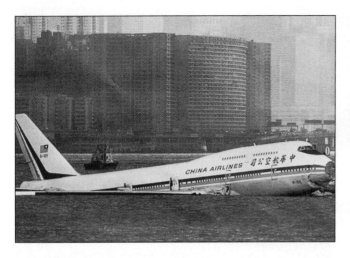
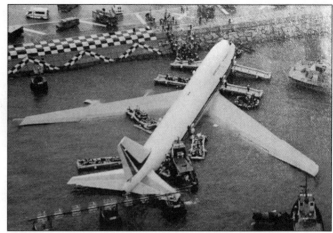

Taiwan's China Airlines is no stranger to spectacular airport arrivals. This is one of their newly delivered 747-400s in Hong Kong harbour some years later.

leaving a cruising altitude is around 2500 feet per minute; a controlled emergency descent after decompression is around 6000 feet per minute. They had greatly exceeded all those figures and survived.

The F/O called Oakland control centre,

"Flight 006... flameout, ah, we emergency... we are niner thousand feet..." Understandably shaken and not speaking in his native language, he got the message across. Oakland had not had a reply to the descent clearance it had relayed to them just as the crisis erupted; they had called several times since. They knew nothing but had suspected the worst, they were very glad to hear from the flight again and that it was stabilised, albeit at a slightly different altitude than when they last communicated!

The crew found that the Engineer's analysis that the other three engines had failed was incorrect, it turned out to be erroneous instrument readings due to their unusual attitudes and speed. They were back under control and had power. The F/E had even been able to successfully restart the rogue number four engine. It was decided to resume their flight to Los Angeles!

The F/O requested radar vectors to get them back on course and a climb to a more fuel efficient altitude. Oakland cleared them to FL 200 and offered them a diversion to San Francisco which was much closer than Los Angeles.

"Condition normal now" replied Flight 006 and declined the offer of the San Francisco diversion.

Everything was still far from normal however. As they climbed further to FL 350 to continue their flight the F/E noticed a number of warning lights on his panel indicating that the body gear of the aircraft was down and locked and that the gear doors were still open, abnormal in itself. Coupled with an apparent total loss of hydraulic fluid in one of the four hydraulic systems something was very amiss. They stopped their climb and did some calculations. If the gear was down and the doors open it would considerably raise their fuel consumption, San Francisco was much closer, that airport suddenly became a very attractive option. The Captain instructed the F/O to tell Oakland that they would divert to San Francisco after all.

Some 20 minutes from San Francisco, due to the abnormalities they were observing they finally decided to declare an emergency. They made their descent and,

lowering the rest of the undercarriage by the manual system since the normal hydraulic system had failed, they made their approach to the left hand of the two westerly runways, 28L. After landing the Captain cleared the runway but, lacking nosewheel steering due to the hydraulic problems, Flight 006 was towed to the arrival gate. They had arrived and the full extent of the effects of their incredible dive became apparent.

Visible to the naked eye, large sections of the extremities of both sides of the tailplane (horizontal stabiliser) had been torn off and there were highly visible puncture marks in the tail area of the fuselage. The engineers went to work to reveal the full extent of the damage.

The Auxiliary Power Unit, a small jet engine mounted in the tail, had broken free from its mounting under the enormous stresses placed on it and had come to rest on part of the fuselage structure. Major components in the undercarriage system had broken free and hydraulic lines to the elevator had been severed causing the loss of hydraulic fluid. The aircraft, even with the large safety factors that Boeing builds in, had never been designed for such abuse.

The flight recorder 'black box' was taken away for analysis and it was found that it too had been adversely affected and had not recorded data for short periods of time. The data that was recovered and readable was amazing. The aircraft had pulled over 5G and had several periods of substantial negative G. The aircraft's performance limits were 2.5G to minus 1.0G!

Every airspeed limitation had been exceeded and, with a limiting Mach number of .92, not far below the speed of sound (Mach 1), it was highly probable that the SP had gone supersonic although the flight recorder was not functioning for the periods that this may have occurred. All of this and yet the airframe had held up and the aircraft had made a safe landing.

Apart from one crewmember who needed hospital treatment, there were no injuries to the crew or passengers undoubtedly thanks to the seatbelt sign fortuitously being on when the upset commenced.

The Boeing 747 had proved to be stronger than anyone imagined and the crew and passengers certainly owed their lives to a company who not only build a wonderful aircraft to fly and fly in, but one that was inadvertently taken far beyond the limits.

CHAPTER FOUR

Flying Blind

The cast of this remarkable story of skill and courage consists of an aircraft carrier, a fighter aircraft, two pilots and a bird, a large one!

The aircraft carrier was HMS *Hermes*, one of the Royal Navy's light fleet carriers. The keel for this vessel was laid in 1944, towards the end of WWII, when it was much needed to replace losses at sea. However, before construction progressed far, the war ended and with it the need for another ship of war – the nation's economy dictated that work was suspended on the vessel.

In the 1950s, defence planning called for several new aircraft carriers and so the project was revived. The shipyards of Vickers-Armstrongs at Barrow in Furness were a hive of activity as the complex structure gradually took shape. There were many modifications to be made to the initial design since the original vessel had been planned for the relatively lightweight piston engined aircraft of the 1940s, now jet fighters were in service in the Royal Navy, heavier and faster than the wartime aircraft.

Completed in late 1959, after undergoing sea trials, she was accepted by the Royal Navy and commissioned. However it was just at this time that yet another generation of naval fighters was being developed and coming into squadron service. These latest aircraft were even bigger and heavier than their predecessors were and they would test the capabilities of the light fleet carriers to the limit. The angled flight deck of the Hermes had been stretched to its maximum to give the longest landing area and angled at 6.5 degrees, it had the greatest angle of any carrier in the fleet.

The Supermarine Scimitar day fighter was a twin engined brute designed to carry a large amount of weaponry as well as missiles. Capable of climbing to great altitudes in less than two minutes she was different to all other naval aircraft for landing.

Most pilots likened landing the Scimitar to a 'controlled crash' often being somewhat ambivalent about the 'controlled' bit. To land it on an airfield the aircraft was not 'flared' to soften the touch down; it was simply flown into the ground. Fortunately it is exactly this technique that is used for carrier landings. Pilots soon got used to the aircraft and found it a pleasure to fly.

Carrier landings require great skill and very accurate flying. If not on centreline the arrester wires will pull out unevenly and the landing aircraft may go 'over the side'. Too fast and the hydraulic jacks providing the stopping power of the arrester wires may bottom out causing the aircraft hook to pull out – the aircraft then trickles off the front of the ship in most cases. Too low and you hit the 'round down' and skittle down the deck in a fiery ball. The only safe error is to be too high and miss all the arrester wires doing a 'bolter'. This usually costs the pilot dearly at the wardroom bar later!

When the weather is bad and there is a heavy swell running it toughens up the task considerably. The deck can be pitching up and down 20 feet or more and, in a cross swell, the whole ship 'corkscrews' making the task of hitting the centreline a chancy business.

The British developed 'mirror landing sight' – which replaced the Landing Signals Officer or 'batsman' as he was popularly known – was an invention that greatly assisted accurate landings. It could be adjusted to target a specific arrester wire and to vary the height of the approaching aircraft over the round down, very important when the ship was heaving. The magnitude of the achievement of Lt Mike Tristram can be better judged with these facts in mind.

It was the 14 July 1962. HMS *Hermes* was conducting exercises to the west of the Mediterranean island of Crete. The Scimitars of 803 Squadron were launching for another sortie, the second of that day. Parked in ranks on the flightdeck, they started their engines on the command from 'flyco', the ship heeled as it turned into wind and a violent shuddering was noticeable as the twin Parsons geared turbines powered the ship to maximum speed for the launch. Flag foxtrot was run up the signal halyards – flying operations were now in progress.

The shattered glass and remains of the bird struck his face and the full force of the 480 knot gale now coming straight at him threw him into a corner of the cockpit despite the tightly fastened safety harness.

The aircraft taxied forward to the twin steam catapults and were loaded on, the launch 'strop', which would fall away after take off, was fitted to the underside of each fighter. The launch officer waved his flag vigorously in a circular motion signalling the pilot to apply full power. The engine screamed and the crackling roar of the raw power could be felt throughout the body. Having checked the engine instruments, the pilot briefly raised one hand showing he was ready for launch. With his right hand on the control column, the elbow jammed into his waist to counter the high G acceleration, and the other hand flat against the back of the throttles, he braced against his ejector seat. The flag dropped and a brief second later, the catapult fired accelerating the 17 tonne aircraft to flying speed in just over one second. It was spectacular to watch and an adrenaline rush for the pilot.

Mike Tristram and his wingman Sub Lt Ben Bosworth launched safely and joined up in battle formation to proceed to the exercise area over Crete. They were directed to their target by the Airborne Early Warning twin

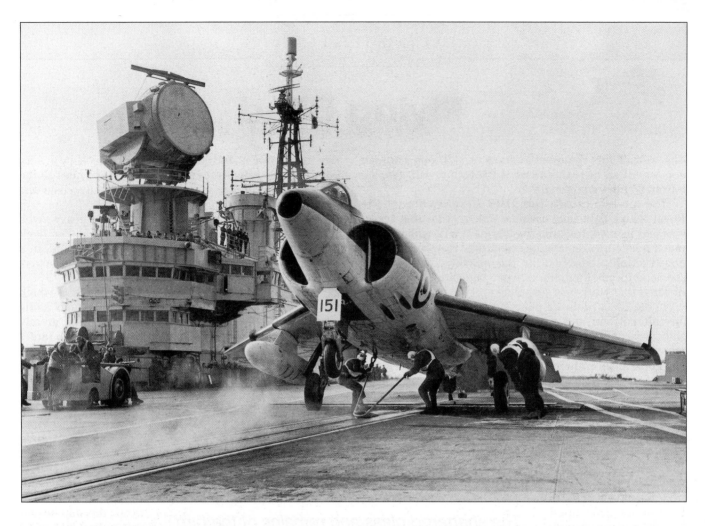

A Supermarine Scimitar preparing to launch from a Royal Navy carrier, note the catapult being connected to the aircraft. (Royal Navy)

engined Gannet aircraft which had been launched earlier and was already 'on station'. They were to carry a simulated Bullpup missile strike on an airfield near the town of Timbakion. Ben Bosworth, whose Scimitar was also equipped for high speed aerial photography, would do the photographic run to record the damage for the intelligence officers back on the ship.

Both aircraft swept in; Mike Tristram in the lead 'fired' the simulated missile while Ben Bosworth dropped down, cameras running 'covered' by his leader above. The photographic run completed they turned to join up at 3000 feet for the quick return to the ship. Mike seeing him approach and realising that they were running a little late for their scheduled land on time, added power to increase their speed to 480 knots (552mph or 889kph).

Ben had not yet resumed battle formation and Mike glanced back to ensure that his wingman would still be able to catch up – it was important that they travelled as one unit in close formation. As he turned once more to scan the horizon for the ship he had a fleeting impression of a large bird, believed to be an eagle, immediately in front of his aircraft. That was the last thing he saw clearly before he was smashed into unconsciousness as the bird struck the front windscreen, passing right through nearly two inches of specially toughened glass and perspex. The shattered glass and remains of the bird struck his face and the full force of the 480 knot gale

now coming straight at him threw him into a corner of the cockpit despite the tightly fastened safety harness.

It is not clear how long he was unconscious – no crewmembers to witness the incident close up and no cockpit recorders on this aircraft – but after a while he came round. He could not understand why he couldn't see anything nor why he was in such a peculiar position hunched in the right hand corner of the tiny cockpit but he did remember seeing the bird and wondered if it had come through the windscreen.

Dismissing this as improbable since he would certainly have been killed in that event, he sat up straight to 'sort things out', a brief and very unsuccessful idea. He immediately felt the full force of the 480 knot windblast coming straight through his shattered front windscreen and was once again thrown violently backwards. It was then that he realised that the bird had come right through his front windscreen and decided that 'cowering to the side of the cockpit' was a good idea!

He then set about trying to regain some vision. The cockpit was full of the remains of the bird, blood, guts and entrails, bone and so on. A revolting and bloody mess. He started to claw away at the debris but, as he thought at the time, he was not sure how much was bird and how much the remains of his face. The entrails felt ominous and, in his dazed state, he thought his skull had been split open and that his brains were now spilling down his face.

His efforts met with a small measure of success. He could now just distinguish between the relative dark of the inside of the cockpit and the bright Mediterranean sky outside. He waggled the wings of his aircraft to call his wingman up into close formation so he too could assess the damage and, having seen the problem, provide much needed assistance. He also slowed the aircraft to reduce the terrifying battering from the windblast from which it was almost impossible to shelter.

Ben Bosworth crept slowly into close formation and saw something red splattered all over the remaining cockpit canopy, it looked like red hydraulic fluid but what was hydraulic fluid doing in the cockpit? He knew his leader was in trouble but, unable to see the shattered front windscreen of Mike's aircraft, he was totally mystified and had no idea of the severity of the emergency, merely stayed close with him awaiting his call on the radio.

Mike was still clearing away the ghastly mess from his face, each time getting faint glimmers of light which immediately dimmed again as more blood flowed into his damaged eyes. He called his wingman on the radio to tell him the full extent of his predicament and to get assistance maintaining altitude and the heading for the ship.

His occasional and minimal vision did not extend to any sight of his vital instruments. The radio microphone, situated in the oxygen mask worn at all times during flight, had also sustained damage as it was struck by the implosion. Mike's transmissions were mostly unreadable although he was not aware of this. His reception of other radio calls, despite the incredible wind noise in the cockpit, was good and he could not understand why he was not getting the assistance he so desperately needed. He finally managed to radio to his wingman that he was disabled and that he needed a 'running commentary' to keep him from crashing into the sea and to get him back at least near to the ship.

Ben was now faced with a most difficult task. Normally the formation leader calls the shots, not having to concentrate on formatting, he can check his instruments for speed and heading and controls the formation. Ben was the wingman to a leader whose flying was unpredictable and occasionally erratic and he still did not know the full extent of the problem. He not only had to ensure that his formation flying was accurate but had to carry out the leader's role as well and get them both back to the ship, it tested all his skills.

At this stage Mike had not even considered how he was going to get back on board. His initial thoughts were to get back close to the ship and eject so that he could be quickly picked up by the rescue 'chopper' but he was uncertain if the ejection seat had also been damaged and whether it would function. The canopy could have also been damaged, would it jettison allowing him to eject? It was possible to eject through the canopy but although

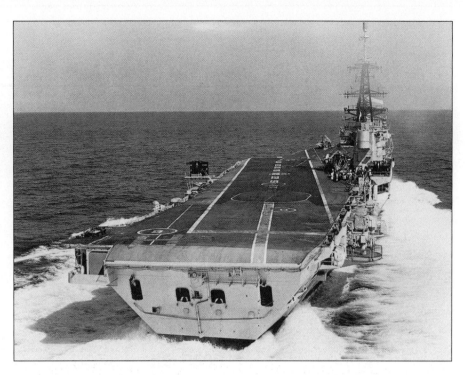

HMAS Hermes *at sea, in a later and much modified form this carrier served in the 1982 Falklands campaign before being later sold to India as INS* Viraat. *This is the view a pilot has during his final seconds prior to landing aboard. Imagine doing this blind, solely following the directions of your wingman! (Royal Navy)*

this was a commonplace emergency escape method in earlier aircraft, trials of such a desperate measure on the Scimitar were far from complete or satisfactory.

The possibility of returning to Crete and landing on an airfield had passed his mind but they had had no briefing of airfields which could accept them. The prospect of the longer flight to an unknown airfield and the uncertainty that immediate and expert medical care would be available was not inviting. He dismissed that alternative. He would be in good hands in the sickbay of HMS *Hermes* much sooner if he pressed on back to the ship.

Either the flow of blood was diminishing or his 'clearance technique' was improving. Mike could now get glimpses of major features and dimly see the horizon but was totally reliant on his wingman for directions and advice on his aircraft's performance, he still could not see a single instrument in his cockpit.

On board the ship they had become aware that one of their aircraft was in trouble but no idea of the extent of the problem. They prepared for an emergency landing. The Commander Air, however, seemed to have a better grasp of the facts and decided that a blind landing back on board was far too dangerous. There was every chance that other aircraft on deck could be damaged and even if they cleared the flightdeck of personnel there was no telling where or how the aircraft would arrive.

Many pilots in the past, in less traumatic circumstances, have flown into the 'island', the multi-deck superstructure on the right hand side of the flightdeck. He ordered Mike to eject but Mike cannot recollect ever receiving this order. In his traumatised state, coupled with the lingering doubts concerning the serviceability of his ejection seat, it is quite probable that he had developed 'selective hearing' – Commander Air never fully believed that Mike had not heard this order! Other flight

● <u>Thrilling</u> series about the silent heroes of the Fleet Air Arm

BLINDED PILOT'S FIGHT TO LAND HIS PLANE

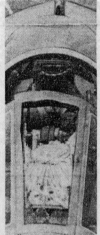

LIEUT. TRISTRAM —A pilot in another fighter acted as "his eyes."

THE large white bird wheeled lazily in the warm air off the south coast of Crete. Just a few miles away Lieutenant Ninian Tristram put his Scimitar jet into a diving attack on Timbakien airfield.

For the 26-year-old pilot this simple exercise in attack was about to turn into a desperate struggle for survival.

The plane and the bird collided. It was, in aviation jargon, a "bird-strike." But one so serious that a few pounds of feathers and flesh nearly knocked a 16-ton Fleet Air Arm fighter out of the sky.

The bird could have hit an engine. The Scimitar would have flown quite happily on the other one.

It could have punched a hole in the skin of the plane. The fighter would have got back to its carrier, H.M.S. Hermes, without too much difficulty.

But no. The bird had to strike the very heart of the aircraft. The pilot!

Lieutenant Tristram first saw it when it was dead ahead of him. Evasive action was impossible.

Crash! The Scimitar and bird collided at a speed of 480 knots. No marksman's bullet could have been deadlier. The bird struck the narrow slit of glass sticking out of the whale-like back of the twin-jet fighter.

Stunned

The front windscreen exploded with the force of the impact. Glass and the shattered remains of the bird struck Ninian Tristram full in the face.

The terrific blow momentarily stunned him. But before the powerful fighter could get out of control he recovered his senses.

And so, on July 14, 1962, Lieutenant N. M. Tristram, of 803 Squadron, found himself in a most bizarre situation.

He was flying his plane, but couldn't see.

His face was cut. There was glass in his eyes. He was covered in blood. And the full force of a 480-knot slipstream was hitting him through the broken panel.

He forced his eyelids open against the wind pressure. Everything was a blur.

A near-blind man was now in control of a bucking monster. The sophisticated aids to flying were useless. He could not see them. And without the aid of the instruments he could not possibly determine the position of the aircraft in the sky, where he was heading, or even which way up he was.

Rapidly his mind ranged over the possibilities.

Just keeping the aircraft straight and level would be difficult enough. But an attempt at landing on Hermes, steaming off the coast of Crete, seemed right out of the question.

He could eject. But, then, £500,000 of aircraft would go spinning into a thousand pieces.

Instead, the man from Ayr put out the call that electrifies all who receive it. "Mayday, Mayday, Mayday" —the international code of distress—went out over the air.

Red blur

The parent ship heard it. And so did Sub-Lieutenant Bosworth, of Weston-Super-Mare, Tristram's wingman. Over the radio came Bosworth's comforting voice acknowledging he was close at hand.

The sub-lieutenant edged his Scimitar closer—and groaned in dismay. The cockpit of the stricken aircraft was stained red. All he could see "was a red blur, which appeared to be Lieutenant Tristram's head."

The injured pilot put the question to him. Am I flying straight and level? Bosworth confirmed that the Scimitar was flying beautifully.

This gave Ninian Tristram time to wipe the blood from his head. Most of it had come from the bird—but some was oozing from cuts in the face. Every move was an effort as the slipstream flattened him to the seat.

Slowly he reduced speed to lessen the wind force. Blinking his eyelids rapidly and ducking to one side of the cockpit, he looked to where the attitude indicator should be. He could just see a hazy outline of the instrument.

Good. It showed he was reasonably straight and level, still in some sort of command of his aircraft.

But setting course for the carrier was another matter.

In a head-on collision a bird nearly knocked a 16-ton aircraft out of the sky

It would take some doing. Still, with Sub-Lieutenant Bosworth as his "guide dog" he might just manage the tricky operation.

Lieutenant Tristram put his thoughts into words over the radio. The pilot in the plane alongside agreed it was the only way out. His eyes, his instruments, would have to be used to fly both of the Scimitars.

He gave his instructions. "Left, left, steady." Like a puppet responding to invisible strands of radio

Below—the cause of it all . . . or what is left of it!

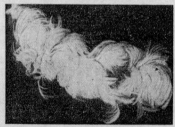

waves, Lieutenant Tristram eased his controls in answer to Bosworth's orders.

Minutes seemed like hours until two planes, as if tied together by a piece of string, thundered over the aircraft carrier.

The crucial moment had arrived. Whether to make an attempt at a landing or to eject.

Just then Tristram caught a glimpse of the ship's wake.

His pulse quickened at the thought that full sight was returning. But his eyes, thick with glass, blood and wind, were in no condition for him to make a spot-on landing without outside assistance.

He could see a little—but could not really focus his eyes. The huge carrier was just a grey blur.

He decided to have a go.

A gamble

The other plane was still flying alongside keeping up a running commentary on their position. Bosworth would have to talk the crippled Scimitar round on the landing circuit and, on the final approach, hand over control to the ship.

The two men started the great gamble. They went through the landing procedure as if Siamese twins. Flaps down! Check. Under-carriage down! Check. Arresting hook lowered! Check.

Tristram began the

On the right—the Scimitar's shattered cockpit.

approach that would eventually take him on to the flight deck of the Hermes.

But there was a big complication. He would not be able to see the landing mirror.

This is a device which has proved a godsend to modern pilots. It indicates they are at the right angle to make a landing.

The mirror reflects a ball of light. When this is level with a line of green lights the aircraft is on the correct landing path.

But to the half-blind Tristram it was now as much use as an ordinary mirror hanging over a mantelpiece.

He could not even see the mirror—let alone the ball of light!

The officer in control of the mirror took over the "duties" of this landing aid. He carefully sighted a telescope attached to the landing mirror on to the aircraft. A calibrated scale on the telescope gave the degree of angle.

The job of being the eyes of Lieutenant Tristram had now passed from Sub-Lieutenant Bosworth to the Mirror Control Officer.

Too low

Reduced to landing speed, the Scimitar came slowly towards the stern of the Hermes.

The Mirror Control Officer focussed the telescope on to the aircraft and read off the angle of approach.

Into his microphone he poured a stream of instructions to the injured pilot. Too high. Down, down. Steady. Left, left. Right, right. Steady.

To every command, Lieutenant Tristram responded with slight movements of his control column. The ship was still a blur. He had to rely entirely on the Mirror Control Officer to get him down.

But everything seemed to be going along fine.

Then, suddenly, a heart-lurching instruction. You are too low! Overshoot.

It would mean carrying on over the aircraft carrier to make another landing attempt.

Tristram's hand quickly reacted to the warning. He pushed the throttle open. The twin jets responded and gave the power needed to go round again.

But at the very moment his aircraft clawed for altitude he caught a well-defined glimpse of the flight deck through the port quarter panel. It was now or never.

Safe landing

He eased back on the throttle. The roar of the engines turned to a whisper. The fighter sank down to the flight deck.

This was not the time for the hook to miss the arresting wires. If it did, a ditching was inevitable.

With a sigh of relief, he felt the comforting jerk as the hook found a wire.

He was down.

The skill and nerve to put himself in the hands of two other men had paid off.

Later the remains of the bird were found in the cockpit. Its identity became the topic of conversation in the carrier. Lieutenant Tristram, who soon recovered from his injuries, believed it to be an eagle.

He was awarded the Queens commendation for his brave conduct.

Next Week—A pilot was lying seriously injured in Communist-held territory and had to be rescued at all costs.

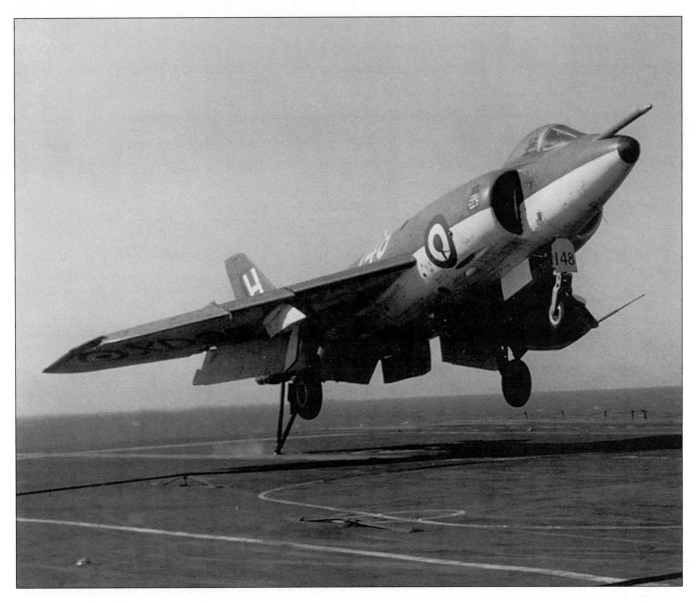

A Scimitar about to catch the across deck tripwire with its arrestor hook. Note the high angle of attack on approach, which limits the pilot's forward vision at the best of times and is just another reason why landing aboard a carrier is about the most challenging task required of any aviator. (Royal Navy)

staff, apparently unaware of the order to eject, continued to prepare for the arrival of an aircraft in distress.

As his wingman shepherded him skilfully towards the carrier Mike was able to make out the foaming white wake of the ship and decided that if he "aimed just ahead of the wake" he might see enough of the ship to pull off a successful landing. In the cold light of day this very inaccurate approximation of how the approach to the tiny deck was to be conducted is quite frightening but if he missed all the wires there was still the option of adding full power, pulling up and attempting an ejection hoping the seat would still do the job for which it was designed. All was now ready on the deck for the landing but, still unaware of what was taking place in the aircraft, they had not rigged the 'crash barrier', designed to rapidly stop any aircraft in an emergency which missed all the wires or had lost its hook. In the circumstances this was a serious, but perhaps fortuitous omission.

Mike had called and asked for a pilot to man the station at the mirror landing sight to give him a running commentary on his approach path, he needed a pilot's view of the approach not that of a technician. The mirror

was still manned by the non-aviator as he started his approach. He regretted the fact that they no longer had an LSO (always a squadron pilot in the days before the mirror sight) who could provide a comforting and expert commentary on his approach and judge the speed of his approach solely from the attitude of the aircraft.

Ben Bosworth, by flying close on his wing, gave him the much needed commentary on his approach path continually calling minute adjustments to his heading and rate of descent to keep him aimed directly at the arrester wires and on centreline. The Mirror Control Officer gave his commentary whenever the approaching Scimitar appeared high or low and interspersed those comments with a 'roger' – you're on the right approach path. Mike was determined that he would 'catch a wire' and bore on down placing his trust in the advice he was receiving.

With only restricted and constantly varying vision he started to make out the dark shadow of the ship beyond the boiling white wake. He was getting close. The directions from his wingman were staccato and to the point but soon he would have to break away, the mirror control officer would have to make all the necessary

APPENDIX "C"

S. 1205C

A list of all accidents, and commendations are to be entered in chronological order as follows :—

(*a*) Brief description of ALL accidents in BLACK ink ;

(*b*) to be followed, where applicable, by commendation in GREEN ink.

(*c*) Where no accident was caused, commendation briefly describing incident is to be entered below in GREEN ink.

	DATE
<u>Serial No. 1.</u>	14th July 1962

On returning from a sortie over Crete, Lieutenant Tristram's aircraft was hit in the front windscreen by a large bird which penetrated both the windscreen and the bullet-proof panel, hitting the pilot in the face and covering him with blood, glass, feathers, entrails and the full force of the slipstream at 480 kts.

Although dazed, injured, temporarily blinded and covered with blood Lieutenant Tristram with the assistance and advice of his No.2, Sub-Lieutenant Bosworth, stayed with his aircraft, maintained control of it, and after recovering sufficiently to have some limited vision, made a safe landing

APPENDIX " C " (continued)

	DATE

on board under most difficult and frightening conditions.

J. Do Ruin

Captain Royal Navy,
Commanding Officer,
H.M.S. Hermes.

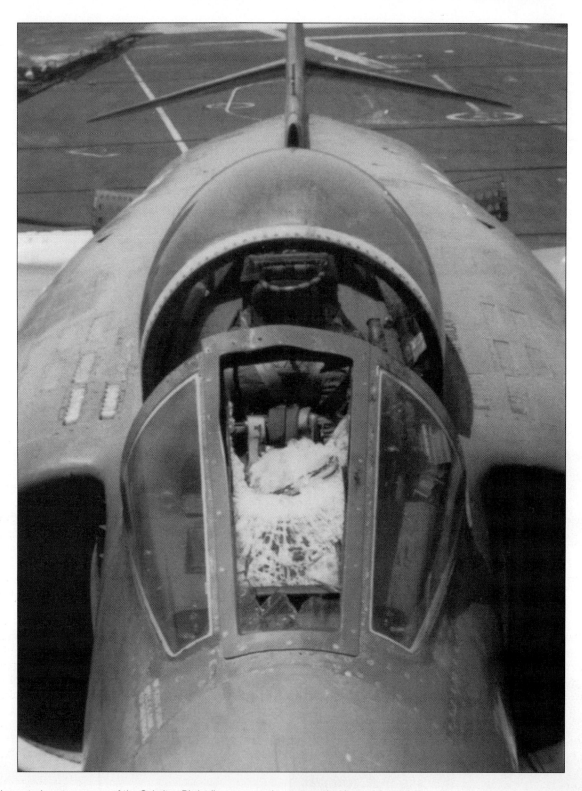

The bird impacted centre screen of the Scimitar. Birdstrikes are a major aeronautical hazard for all forms of aviation and are particularly dangerous for military strike aircraft which spend much of the life at low level and at relatively high speeds. Australia's RAAF lost an F-111 and its two man crew to a birdstrike while the RAF lost a Nimrod four engine long range maritime patrol aircraft and its entire crew when on takeoff from its Cornwall base its engines ingested several dozen large seabirds. (Royal Navy)

corrections for the critical last bit of the approach. Mike's confidence built but he had to keep it up until he felt the aircraft impact with the deck and the deceleration as the aircraft hook engaged an arrester wire. If there was no deceleration he was left with no alternative, it had to be an ejection.

At the last minute and to avoid flying into the ship's mast, his wingman peeled off leaving his leader with just a few feet of the approach to complete and less than a

second or two from touchdown. With an almighty thud Mike's Scimitar hit the deck. The landing gear oleos compressed to their full extent cushioning the impact and he was immediately thrown forward against his harness as the aircraft came to a stop in under 100 feet. He had landed and caught a wire – virtually blind.

The events that followed his incredible and successful landing were not what a homecoming hero would expect or deserve. As he later commented, "It

Naval Pay Branch,
Admiralty,
S.W. 1.

By the QUEEN'S Order the name of
Lieutenant Ninian Michael Tristram,
Royal Navy,
was published in the London Gazette on
16th November, 1962,
as commended for brave conduct.
I am charged to record Her Majesty's
high appreciation of the service rendered.

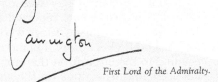

First Lord of the Admiralty.

The enclosed Bronze Oak
Leaf Emblem granted to those
awarded a Queen's Commendation
for Brave Conduct is to be worn
directly on the coat after any
Medal ribands, as laid down in
the Appendix to the Navy List of
June, 1962, page 58. If there
are no Medal ribands, the Emblem
is worn in the position in which
a single riband would be worn.

descended into sheer farce"! The flight deck staff still did not yet comprehend the extent of the problem. Mike raised the hook and folded the wings and started to taxi towards the parking area towards the bow, Fly One in carrier parlance. He had to clear the landing area for his wingman still to land on who would have been in great trouble if he had actually crashed and obstructed the flight deck. He soon realised that his vision did not make it safe to go too far.

Aircraft are parked literally inches from the edge of the deck with the restricted space available. He stopped the aircraft and applied the parking brake but was immediately ordered on the radio to continue to taxy forward and follow the director's instructions to the parking area. What director? There was just a dull blur before him with the flightdeck personnel just amorphous shapes. Taxy and parking directions were simply not visible. It was probably the relief of being on board and shock setting in that caused him to rebel at this stage.

"I've had enough" he thought, "They can find a tractor and tow the thing the last ten yards".

He shut down the engines and the flightdeck crew, seeing that the pilot was in more than a little distress went to his aid. The canopy was firmly jammed, he had been right – an ejection would have been a less than safe option. Crewmen worked on the jammed canopy for several minutes before it was finally opened with a crowbar. Mike started to climb out and asked for assistance to get to the sickbay, his sight so bad that he could not negotiate the ladders and narrow companionways in safety. His thoughts of a soft cot in the sick bay and ministrations of the ship's doctor were rudely dashed.

Now realising that they had an injured pilot destined for the sick bay they planned to treat that as 'an exercise'. He waited whilst an SBA (Sick Berth Attendant)

and a stretcher were brought up on deck and allowed himself to be strapped into the stretcher and lay there under the aircraft waiting. They were going to transport him to the sick bay using the bomb lift which operated between the armoury in the bowels of the ship and the flightdeck via the sickbay level. There was one problem, there was an aircraft parked over the bomb lift and it had to be moved before they could operate the lift to the flight deck. With other aircraft still landing on it was not possible to move the obstructing aircraft.

After a long wait the numbness gradually wore off and pain started to set in and being greatly concerned that he get prompt treatment for the injuries to his eyes, Mike "got a little ratty" and insisted on going to the sickbay immediately. The players in the new 'exercise' reluctantly released him from the stretcher and told him to stand up. He did so and, in his semi-blindness, immediately banged his head sharply on the weapons pylon under the aircraft!

Finally in the sickbay, the delicate and painful task of picking shards of perspex out of his corneas and face commenced. Miraculously none of the shattered windscreen had penetrated far into the eye and his eyesight was not endangered. In the true tradition of 'put them back on the horse' Mike flew again four days later, albeit in a patched up condition with stitches in his face and with somewhat suspect eyesight.

Lt Mike Tristram was awarded the Queen's Commendation for Brave Conduct, a much rarer honour than the more frequently awarded commendation 'For Services in the Air'. He modestly feels that it was his desperate attempts to get quickly to the ship's sickbay rather than bravery that convinced him to attempt the seemingly impossible.

Written and compiled from Lt Tristram's personal account of the incident to the author.

CHAPTER FIVE

Sunset for the 'Funjet'

Some years ago now I was visiting the 'management floor' of my airline after a lengthy period of sick leave when one of the supervisory Captains saw me through his open door.

"Come in John, how are you," he enquired.

I told him that I had recovered from a nasty encounter with hepatitis, possibly picked up abroad, and had come in to get my medical clearance. We chatted for a while when he revealed that the airline had received applications for employment from two women pilots. He was visibly in shock.

"What do you think we should do?" he asked, obviously seeking some means of preventing what he saw as the breaching of the last of the male bastions.

"Why don't you interview them? They might be quite good" I replied. That was the end of our friendly chat!

I am happy to say that the ladies were the first of many to be employed. They proved to be excellent pilots and now command big jets in the company.

The illogical concern exhibited by that management pilot totally ignored the fact that amongst the pioneers of aviation, the ladies featured very strongly. Amelia Earhart, Amy Mollison and Australia's own Nancy Bird Walton to name but a few; their exploits are legendary. Women have been flying professionally as airline pilots for some years now but it was not until 1988 that a woman crewmember was involved in an inflight catastrophe and proved that they can match it with the best.

Aloha Airlines operates services between the idyllic Hawaiian Islands. It is one of the smallest route structures in the world, the network covering only 572 kilometres between the five main islands with most of their flights being less than 30 minutes – just a quick 'up and down'.

Their fleet of Boeing 737 aircraft, which they called 'Funjets", were ideal for the purpose and they were worked hard. After nearly 20 years of service some of the aircraft had achieved the distinction of having the highest number of flights of the worldwide fleet of Boeing 737 aircraft and, as such, had come under the aegis of Boeing's special Aging Fleet Program. This program was devised to constantly evaluate the condition and safety of older or heavily used aircraft made by the Boeing Company in the interests of safety and as a service to their customers.

With their very short sectors, Aloha's aircraft were of particular interest since they performed nearly three times the fleet average number of cycles. A cycle is when an aircraft climbs and is pressurised and then depressurised again on descent. Despite the sig-

Observing that the cockpit door had vanished and through the gap where it had been, there was only blue sky, the Captain immediately took over the controls and commenced an emergency descent.

nificantly heavy use of the Aloha 737s, since they rarely climbed high on their short trips, they did not experience the full wear and tear of aircraft cruising at higher altitudes with greater pressure differentials between the cabin and the outside atmosphere. Even with their high number of cycles, they were regarded as thoroughly airworthy. The certification testing of the 737 involved a fuselage being put through 150,000 cycles, the aircraft on this flight, registered N73711, had completed just over 85,000 cycles.

Another beautiful day was dawning when Captain Robert Schornstheimer reported for duty on April 23 1988. He and his First Officer were to operate six short inter-island flights before a planned change of F/O. Proceeding to the aircraft on the ramp, the F/O carried out his preflight inspections on the aircraft whilst the Captain picked up the flightplan and weather forecasts in the dispatch office. It was all very routine and they successfully completed the six short return flights from Honolulu to Hilo, Maui and Kauai. The planned F/O switch then took place and F/O Madeline Tomkins joined the aircraft.

Captain Schornstheimer was an 11 year veteran with Aloha Airlines and had over 6700 hours experience on the Boeing 737 alone whilst the new F/O had been with Aloha nine years and had over 8000 hours flying experience, 3500 hours of which was also on the 737. They were a highly experienced crew.

The first two flights for the new crew complement were from Honolulu to Maui and then from Maui to Hilo on the Big Island of Hawaii. With the short flights and very short turnarounds, both pilots remained in the cockpit whilst the arriving passengers disembarked and the departing passengers boarded for their flight. They were now Aloha Flight 243 destined for Honolulu with the short cruise planned at Flight Level 240 (24,000 feet).

It was as the passengers were boarding that the first clue to what was about to happen came to light. A female passenger noticed a small crack in the fuselage between the aircraft door and the hood of the aerobridge. Thinking that the crew must have known about it or being reluctant to appear silly, she chose not to mention it to any of the crew. It is interesting, in retrospect to wonder what would have happened had she raised the matter.

"Little old lady says there is a crack in the fuselage"

"Yeah, well tell her to sit down and get strapped in, we're on our way"

Or perhaps it would have been reported to the pilots

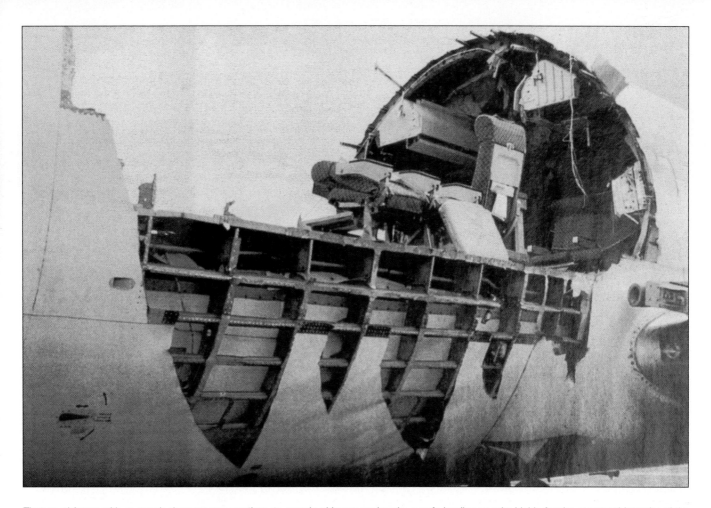

That an airframe with so much damage can continue to remain airborne and make a safe landing speaks highly for the structural integrity of the modern day jetliner. The enemy though is age and corrosion and the latter has been addressed since this landmark accident with a series of monitoring and repair programs put in place for older airliners. In this photo most of the seats have already been cleared away for closer inspection of the structure by Boeing and NTSB engineers. (NTSB)

who may have checked it out and delayed the service for more expert advice. One can only speculate.

With F/O Tomkins operating as the pilot for this leg and the Captain carrying out the support role and making the radio calls, they made a routine departure for Honolulu. It was a fine day with clear weather and Madeline elected to fly the aircraft manually, not engaging the autopilot. Pilots rarely get a chance to practice their skills in this area and take every opportunity to hone their touch on the controls.

Just as the F/O levelled out smoothly at 24,000 feet there was a loud noise followed by what they described as a 'whooshing' sound. Despite wearing her safety harness the F/O was thrown about in her seat and debris floated around the flightdeck. They had experienced an explosive decompression of the aircraft cabin. Both pilots immediately pulled their quick release oxygen masks from their stowages and snapped them on.

It was essential to be breathing pressurised oxygen at what was now a cabin altitude of 24,000 feet. The Captain, observing that the cockpit door had vanished, and through the gap where it had been he could see the sky, immediately took over the controls and commenced an emergency descent. He found that the aircraft was rolling gently left and right and the controls felt far from normal. Some major damage had occurred to the aircraft: they had a critical emergency on their hands.

The noise on the flightdeck was such that the two pilots could not communicate with each other but used hand signals to signify their intents. The aircraft descended rapidly and under full control towards an altitude where crew or passengers would not need oxygen. The F/O carried out the drills in her seat and set the radar transponder code to the emergency setting. Air Traffic Control would know immediately that their aircraft was in an emergency situation, would ensure they had priority and would provide them with every assistance. She called Honolulu on the radio but the noise was such that she could not hear if they replied. She hoped the transponder would tell them all they needed to know.

In the cabin there was total chaos. Luckily, when the decompression occurred, the seat belt sign was still on and the passengers still had their seat belts fastened. The stewardesses though, were moving about the cabin carrying out their normal duties. One girl, Flight Attendant Clarabelle Lansing, the only fatality, was drawn out of the aircraft by the rushing air through a rapidly developing hole in the fuselage. Another, Flight Attendant Jane Sato-Tomita, was hit by flying debris and was now unconscious on the floor with serious head injuries whilst the third Flight Attendant, Michelle Honda, was thrown violently to the floor by the blast of air and sustained severe bruising. All in the cabin were only too aware of the extent of the damage; a large section of the roof and walls of the forward cabin had simply been

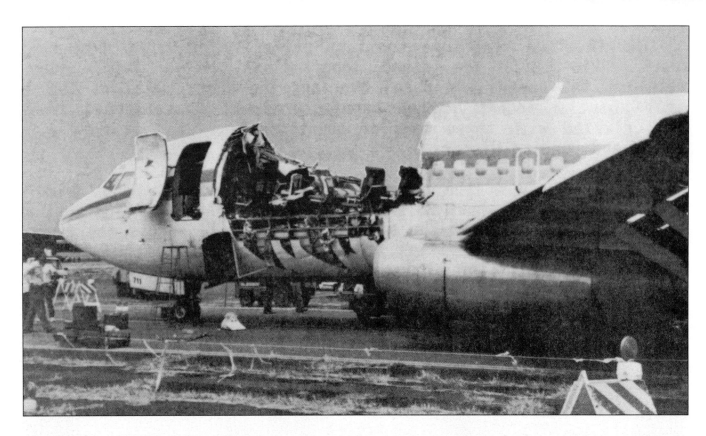

This photo was taken just after the passenger evacuation with the cabin seats remaining in place. The slipstream endured by the more exposed passengers would have at times been in excess of 500kph. (NTSB)

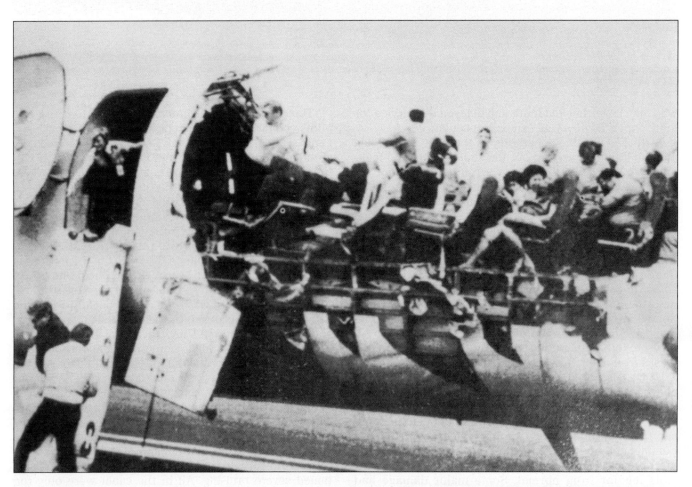

Passengers evacuate via the deployed front door slide assisted by a flight attendant. Other passengers are standing while still others remain seated and injured. (NTSB)

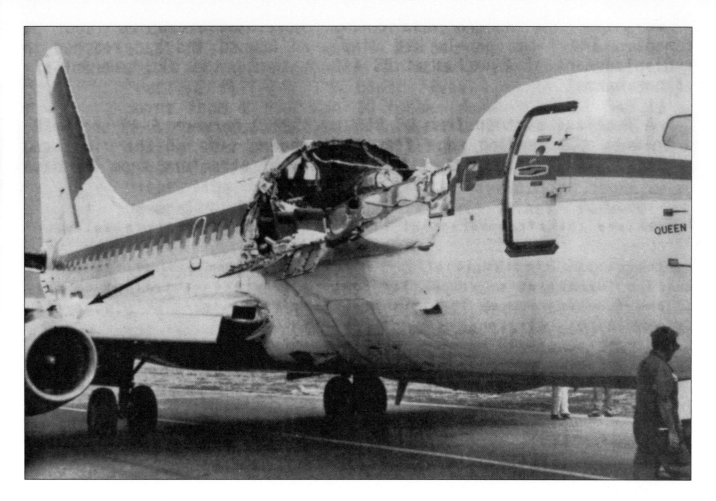

The right side of the 737 tended to have its fuselage roof and side panels peeled outwards while the other side largely had them torn away as the cabin roofing peeled open. (NTSB)

blown away. Amazingly, Michelle Honda bravely crawled up and down the aisle comforting and assisting the terrified passengers many of whom had sustained injuries in the initial decompression. Others were still being injured by the slipstream and turbulent air now entering the severely damaged cabin.

The Air Traffic Controller had not heard the first desperate call from the F/O but he had seen the Mayday 'squawk' from the transponder on his radar screen at a position just 23 miles south-southeast of Maui's Kahalui airport. He tried to contact the aircraft several times without success but, with the 'blip' still on his screen, he knew the aircraft was still flying. He alerted his colleagues to the situation.

As the aircraft passed through 14,000 feet the F/O, knowing that Maui airport was their closest runway, switched her radio to Maui tower frequency and was able to declare an emergency and tell them what little she knew of the problem. She had no knowledge of the problems in the cabin since they had been unable to contact the cabin crew at all. It was obviously very serious though and she stated a need for a full emergency turn out for their arrival. The rescue vehicles now lined the side of the runway to await the arrival of flight 243. Since the flight was still technically out of the area controlled by Maui tower the controller requested a change in transponder code which would inform all that the aircraft was now under the control of Maui tower, albeit beyond his normal area of control

As they approached 10,000 feet the Captain began to slow the aircraft from its high speed descent and, now they were at a safe level, removed his oxygen mask and turned the aircraft towards the north-north-easterly runway 02 at Maui airport. Now there was less wind noise the two pilots could communicate with relative ease and, preparing for a landing, the Captain called for the first flap extension and then for five degrees of flaps. When he requested the next flap extension as the speed reduced he found that control of the aircraft rapidly became more difficult so he reverted to the five degree setting and planned to land in this configuration. Any speed below 170 knots also made control difficult and the decision was made to land at this higher than normal speed. The generous runway length at Maui would still enable them to stop safely.

The F/O coolly went about her duties supporting the Captain. She tried a further communication with the cabin using the public address system but there was no reply. The Captain called for the landing gear to be lowered as they commenced their approach. She pulled the gear lever out of its detent and selected it to the down position. The two main gear lights went green indicating that the main wheels were safely down and locked but there was no green light for the nose gear, nor was there a warning light which would tell them that it hadn't fully lowered. The manual lowering system was operated, but still without success.

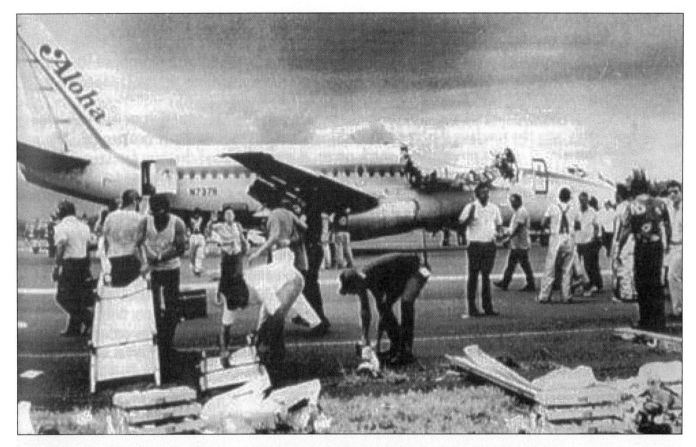

Rescue workers assemble seat cushions and cabin debris prior to the aircraft undergoing intensive inspection by Boeing and NTSB officials. (NTSB)

As far as they knew it would be a 'nose gear up' landing and the need to land as soon as possible made that the lesser of two evils. The Captain asked the F/O to tell the controller "We got such problems but we are going to land anyway – even without the nose gear – but they should be aware that we do not have a safe nose gear indication". The F/O advised the tower of this new crisis and of the Captain's intentions adding "We'll need all the equipment you've got". Those on the ground were now fully aware of the extent of their plight.

The Captain added power to stabilise his approach and the substantial yaw of the aircraft told him that his number one engine had failed. They tried a restart but the engine did not respond. They were now approaching to land with a severely damaged aircraft which was handling strangely, with reduced flap setting, at a higher speed than normal with a possible nose gear failure and with one engine failed. The Captain was also aware of other problems. The aircraft was shaking, rocking slightly and, he said later, felt 'springy'. He did not know it at the time but the damage was so severe that the aircraft was very close to breaking up and the fuselage forward of the damage was bending and drooping over a metre – this was the springy feeling he was getting.

They got their first bit of good news when the tower controller, having a close look at the aircraft through binoculars, advised them that the nose gear appeared to be safely extended. They needed all the good news they could get! The crews of the waiting emergency vehicles watched in amazement as Flight 243 came into their view, the fuselage half gone and with the nose of the aircraft visibly bending as if it were about to snap off completely.

Approximately 13 minutes after the aircraft cabin had disastrously blown out Captain Schornstheimer landed on Maui's runway 02 with what he later described, in a masterpiece of understatement, as 'a normal touchdown'. He used the reverse thrust on the remaining engine to help slow the aircraft and the F/O extended the flaps to the full landing configuration to effect some aerodynamic braking. They came to a safe stop on the runway.

F/O Tomkins left her seat and opened the main cabin door and deployed the escape slide allowing passengers who could move to escape from the remains of the aircraft. It was a sensible move since there was always the chance of further problems. The Captain with Flight Attendant Michelle Honda, who was still able to move about, assisted the mobile passengers to the slides and to the rear airstairs. Rescue crews then boarded and assisted those who were injured and still in their seats. Except for the tragic loss of the stewardess, all crew and passengers survived.

In a severe multiple emergency situation such as this survival hinges on the correct actions of the crew as a whole. The Captain's handling skills and experience had brought the aircraft back but without the vital support of his First Officer it would have been much harder. All crewmembers displayed superb professionalism and great coolness in the face of almost impossible odds.

The thorough and detailed investigation by the US National Transportation Safety Board indicated that the cabin failure could have started just where the passenger had noted a crack. A definitive answer to this was made difficult by the fact that the missing portion of the cabin was never recovered.

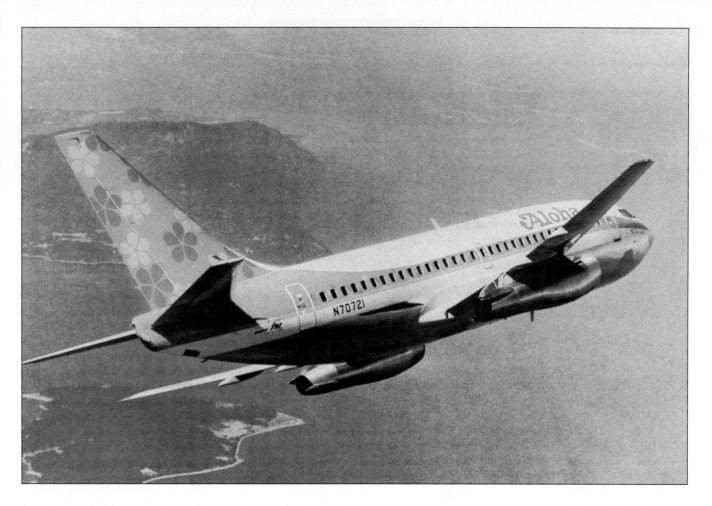

An Aloha 737-100 in happier times. Operating in a semi tropical maritime environment with a very high rate of cycles ultimately led to a near catastrophe that also was a timely wakeup call for the entire airline community worldwide. (Aloha Airlines)

Nonetheless, the extensive recommendations made by the Board of Enquiry and the evidence available from the remains of the fuselage enabled significant improvements to maintenance procedures and other measures to prevent any recurrence of this problem. Every time a major incident occurs the safety of the travelling public is improved over and above its already very high level.

The high cost of purchasing airliners means that much time and money is spent repairing apparently irreparable damage after an incident. In this case the damage was so severe that the $5 million aircraft was scrapped and sold for parts.

CHAPTER SIX

Independence Day

If you remember the days of air travel when you could check in, get a boarding pass and blithely go to the boarding gate without hindrance, you may wonder at the many security obstacles placed in your way today. Metal detectors, baggage searches, physical 'pat downs', photo identification requirements and other checks. You may find them intrusive or simply annoying.

Terrorism and sabotage have however, in recent years, become a significant factor demanding stringent counter measures by governments and airlines all of which cost money and add to the cost of your ticket. Money well spent, as any pilot who has flown with a gun at his head will attest.

Reputable airlines provide training for their crews in handling the hijack situation but the infinite variety of scenarios that can arise make specific training hard to formulate. Each situation has to be handled on a developing basis. The deranged passenger making demands is unpredictable and may, or may not, be able to carry out the threat he or she poses. The political terrorist, often a fanatic and also very unpredictable, will most probably have received training in the systems and cockpit layout of the aircraft under threat. Any false move or attempt by crewmembers to covertly notify authorities can result in the use of firearms or other violence against the crew or passengers; it does not take much to trigger an attack from an unstable & violent terrorist.

A pilot was pistol whipped for possessing an Omega brand watch during one hijack, the terrorist insisting that the Greek letter omega on the watch face was a Zionist symbol! The hijackers may commence to kill without warning to prove that they mean business, this places the crew in an almost impossible situation when authorities will not bow to the hijacker's demands. It takes a special sort of crew to contain the situation.

On June 14 1985, TWA flight 847 was scheduled to operate from Cairo to Athens and then on to Rome where many passengers would connect with TWA's intercontinental flight to the United States. Arriving in Athens the aircraft refuelled while the captain and his crew carried out the preflight checks for the next sector of their journey. The cabin crew received fresh catering supplies and as the cleaners finished their work, set about preparing the cabin to receive the passengers. There was less than one hour on the ground before the Boeing 727 trijet resumed its journey.

At the check-in desk the passengers placed their baggage on the scales and presented their tickets and passports duly receiving their boarding passes – all but one. The young male argued at length with TWA ground staff

"They've just killed a passenger," he shouted to the tower. The hijacker again seized the microphone and screamed, "You see? Now do you believe it?" and threatened another killing in five minutes if the demands weren't met.

and became very unpleasant. This resulted in the ground staff remembering his face very well. An important and significant factor in this tale of tenacity as it would later transpire.

Boarding was complete and Captain John Testrake started the three engines. Checks completed they taxied out for takeoff. Flying in a Boeing 727 was quite eerie, with the engines at the back there was practically no engine noise in the passenger cabin at all. As the Captain applied takeoff thrust, the aircraft seemed to silently accelerate and lift off the ground as if by magic. Immediately after takeoff the aircraft made a left turn out to sea as aircraft were not permitted to fly over the city of Athens. The Captain followed his departure clearance and joined the airway system for the flight to Rome with 145 passengers and eight crew on board.

They had been airborne a little under 20 minutes and were now in Italian airspace when two male passengers got to their feet to visit the toilet. They had been in the toilets only a short time when they emerged again brandishing 9mm pistols and carrying grenades. They swaggered down the centre aisle with loud and hysterical shouts of "Get down, get down, put your heads between your knees" indicating with their pistols that they wanted all passengers to crouch over in their seats.

Those who were not quick enough or who did not crouch low enough for their satisfaction were savagely struck and beaten. The cabin crew stopped their duties and rapidly seated themselves and crouched low in a position they had learnt as the 'brace' position, normally used for emergency landings. These were terrorists in the very real sense of the word.

With the passengers now subdued one hijacker remained in the cabin threatening any passenger who lifted their head with his pistol whilst the other went to the flightdeck – the pilots and engineer were not yet aware of the drama in the cabin. Bursting through the cockpit door, gun and grenade plainly visible, he ordered Captain Testrake to fly the aircraft to Beirut. TWA Flight 847 was under hijack.

First Officer Phillip Maresca did not need a prompt, he could see the gun pointed directly at the Captain's head and the grenade in the terrorist's other hand. He did not want to audibly inform the Italian Air Traffic Control that the flight had been hijacked but he had to get a clearance to the new destination, one wrong word could trigger off a violent reaction from the obviously irrational and stressed hijacker. Phrasing the clearance request with great diplomacy he persuaded the controller that Flight 847 was diverting to Beirut and duly got the

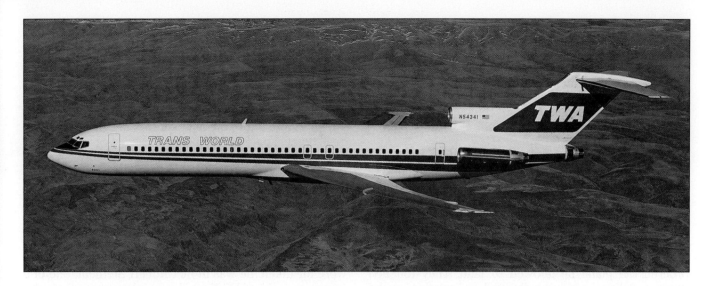

A Tran World Airways Boeing 727-200 the same as, though in a different livery, to the one depicted in this chapter. (Boeing)

necessary clearance. The aircraft turned back and headed east along the airway system. It soon became clear to the ground authorities that the crew were acting under duress and there could only be one reason for that. There had already been two hijacks in the region that week – the word was forwarded on that TWA 847 had been hijacked; now it was out in the open.

As they approached Beirut the First Officer switched radio frequencies to Beirut control and called for a final clearance to the airport. Their situation immediately became more precarious. Whilst under international conventions any aircraft in distress should be given every assistance and their requests immediately granted, no state or airport wants an aircraft under hijack on its soil.

Beirut airport authorities, aware of the imminent arrival, had closed the airport by blocking the runway with buses and other vehicles. Flight 847 was refused permission to land nor could they attempt to land in safety with vehicles on the runway. Captain Testrake was in an extremely difficult situation. He had an armed and desperate hijacker holding a loaded gun and a hand grenade in his cockpit and he could not comply with his demands. There could only be one outcome if Beirut did not open the airport for their arrival. The hijacker in the cockpit hearing that the Beirut runway was closed became increasing threatening. Captain Testrake knew that such fanatics did not care if they lived or died. He did, and he had the lives of all on board in his hands. He argued desperately with the tower.

"We must land, they are beating up the passengers. He has pulled the pin on the grenade, he is going to blow up the plane."

The urgency in the Captain's voice and the prospect of being responsible for the aircraft exploding over Lebanese territory with terrible loss of life finally swayed them and the runway was cleared. Flight 847 landed and was directed to a remote parking area.

Back at Athens the irate passenger who had not been able to board had been arrested and with the subsequent turn of events, was closely interrogated by the Greek police. He had been in the company of two other young men of Lebanese appearance. He was identified as Ali Atweh and admitted that he was one of three terrorists planning to hijack Flight 843 which explained his agitation when refused boarding. He identified the two hijackers on board as Ahmed Gharbiyeh and Ali Youness and that they were members of the Islamic Jihad, a fanatical Muslim fundamentalist group noted for their violent actions against the West.

He claimed that the weapons had been smuggled through the Athens security by wrapping them up in material which they thought would conceal them from the x-ray check. This was highly unlikely. Although Athens security was not highly regarded, it would have been virtually impossible for the weapons to pass through undetected. It was more probable that an accomplice with access to the aircraft had concealed the weapons on board prior to the hijack, possibly in Cairo or even that day in Athens. It mattered not, the weapons were on board and were real and loaded!

As soon as they arrived at Beirut the hijackers announced their demands: the release of several hundred Shiite Muslim prisoners held by the Israeli government in exchange for the lives of all on board. As a sign of good faith they permitted 19 women and children to leave the aircraft. To prevent any potential rescuers gaining easy access to the aircraft these passengers were sent down the emergency escape 'chute which was deployed from the front door of the aircraft. Under a threat to kill passengers and stating that the plane had been 'booby trapped' they demanded that the aircraft be fully refuelled immediately and threatened to blow up the plane if any rescue was attempted during refuelling.

A recent hijack had been ended when military specialists had boarded a hijacked aircraft disguised as mechanics and had overcome the hijackers – they were obviously aware of that incident. They also demanded to talk to an official of the Amal, another Shiite Muslim group, but the Amal officials refused. Not being in control of the situation and with the possible unwanted political implications of this terrorist strike it served Amal's purpose to distance themselves from it at the moment. The turbulent religious and political atmosphere of the Middle East was already complicating the task of the crew who were totally at the mercy of violent and dangerous men.

The refuelling carried out without incident, the hijackers demanded to be flown to Algiers. The aircraft departed Beirut and the authorities, all now well aware of the situation, gave Flight 847 free passage down the airways over the Mediterranean. As they flew the wires were humming around the world as President Reagan and his experts went into conference seeking a peaceful resolution to the hijack. With the crew and passengers under constant threat there was little chance of a military solution without loss of life.

Algiers might be the answer, they could possibly be persuaded to 'sweet talk' the hijackers into surrendering and releasing the hostages as they had done successfully during the American Embassy hostage crisis in Iran not so long ago. It was not an auspicious start when, approaching Algiers, the authorities also closed the airport but a message from President Reagan had already reached the Algerian President Chadli Benjedid and he ordered the plane be allowed to land. They touched down at 3.30pm and were directed to park out on the runway.

Safely on the ground the two hijackers repeated their demands and again had the aircraft refuelled, Captain Testrake's hopes that the flight was over were dashed but another 21 passengers, mostly women and children, were released, that was a good sign if there was one in the circumstances. Undoubtedly he was seething with anger inside but he had to maintain a calm and conciliatory demeanour and counselled his crew to do likewise. Just five hours later the hijackers demanded that the aircraft return to Beirut.

Captain Testrake could only wonder at how long this would go on. The 727 was a 'short haul' aircraft, there was no provision for real crew rest and before long they would all need to get some sleep. The only options were to rest in one of the more comfortable first class seats or try to stretch out across the economy seats now that there were fewer passengers on board. With the constant harassment and shouting from their captors, good rest would be hard to come by, yet he and his crew had to continue to fly the aircraft safely at their captors' behest until a resolution to the hijack was reached. It was going to need great fortitude and no little courage to keep going.

After another flight across the Mediterranean back to Beirut, they were again greeted with the closure of the airport. Captain Testrake was getting a distinct feeling of déja vu! He urgently told the tower that they had little fuel remaining, which was true, and he was under threat of being shot if he did not land at Beirut. Finally one of the hijackers seized the microphone and screamed at the tower operator that if they were not permitted to land they would crash the aircraft into the control tower or even the presidential palace, adding that they were "Suicide terrorists".

The tower controller relented and permitted the aircraft to land once more. It was now well past midnight and the whole crew was dog-tired, they were well past their normal tour of duty. Unbeknownst to the captain, the heavily armed Amal militia was now in control of the airport.

Another demand to have an Amal official come to the aircraft went unheeded. The hijackers promptly seized a male American passenger, hustled him to the open front door and shot him, throwing his body onto the tarmac. The Captain desperately called the tower; he had to ensure that the hijacker's demands were met before further murders took place,

"They've just killed a passenger," he shouted to the tower. The hijacker again seized the microphone and screamed, "You see? Now do you believe it?" and threatened another killing in five minutes if the demands weren't met. The tower tried to remonstrate with him as a fellow Arab but to the hijacker that meant nothing and he screamed back on the radio,

"Did you forget the Bir al Abed massacre?" (A car bombing in Beirut that they wrongly attributed to the CIA that killed more than 75 Shiite Muslims but had missed the main target). If Captain Testrake had had any doubts about the intent of the hijackers, these had quickly evaporated. It turned out that they thought the man they had murdered was an American Marine involved in actions against their cause in Lebanon. They were mistaken, he was in fact Robert Stethem, one of a four man team of US Navy divers who was sadly in the wrong place at the wrong time.

The killing brought results; the Amal official to whom they had been demanding to speak came to the aircraft and talked to the hijackers. While these negotiations took place another demand was issued. All airport lights had to be extinguished. With the killing still very fresh in their minds, the tower complied. The airport was in total darkness.

In the cabin one of the stewardesses was ordered to identify passengers who had Jewish sounding names. The obvious follow up to this action was repugnant to her and she refused but under severe threats she finally had to give in. As they proceeded along the cabin she constantly denied that passengers with certain names were Jewish pointing out that it was a German or other foreign name, not Jewish. She did so at risk of her life. Finally a number of passengers that the hijackers decided were Jewish were hustled off the 'plane to an unknown fate and destination. They were freed from the aircraft but would be kept prisoner for more than a week in a secret location in Beirut.

There were not only people disembarking. Under the cover of darkness a large number of Amal militia came on board bringing with them more weapons and ammunition. Not unsympathetic to the demands of the hijackers, they were an unwelcome addition to the hysterical duo. Any hope that the two hijackers alone would eventually tire and could be overpowered now vanished.

The hijackers called the tower and told them that the Red Cross could come and remove the body of the shot passenger. It had been lying on the tarmac for over two hours. They demanded more fuel and a very specific order of food; the fuel had to come first. Obviously the saga was far from over, the Captain was told they would depart at first light and he called the tower to tell them to have the runway cleared for his dawn departure.

"What will your destination be?" Asked the tower.

"I don't know," was the weary reply. There was time for just a brief sleep before they would takeoff again.

The hijackers made another demand, their colleague who had not boarded in Athens, Ali Atweh, must be released and flown to their nominated destination or they would kill all passengers of Greek nationality. The Greek authorities immediately complied and Atweh was put on an Olympic Airway 'plane and promptly flown to Algiers.

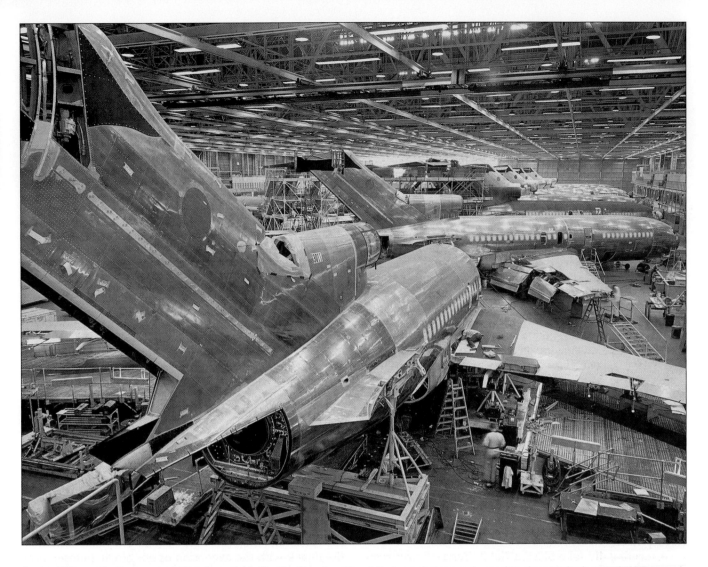

Boeing 727s on the Renton production line outside Seattle. The aircraft's relatively modest range, by modern day standards, acted as an asset in preventing the hijackers ranging further than they did. (Boeing)

At dawn the exhausted crew once again started the engines and was told to return to Algiers. They touched down at 7.30am. About two hours later the hijackers inexplicably released three more passengers, later releasing the Greek passengers in exchange for Atweh who had arrived earlier at Algiers. Thankfully the worldwide diplomatic efforts had paid off and two Algerian officials boarded the aircraft to conduct negotiations for the release of the hostages and aircraft.

All day long the talks with the hijackers continued on the aircraft. The efforts of the Algerians proved fruitful as later in the day another large batch of passengers was allowed to leave the aircraft. They were more than glad to get off. One of the two original hijackers proved to be sadistic and delighted in walking up and down the cabin hitting passengers on the head. Stewardess Uli Derickson, at great personal risk challenged him pointing out that the passengers were complying with his demands so why was he continually beating them up? She was lucky not to be seriously assaulted; it was a very brave act. Other cabin crewmembers acted with equal courage as they tried to protect 'their' passengers.

It was late in the evening when a five man specialist negotiating team arrived from the Red Cross headquarters in Geneva. They continued to attempt to solve the deadly impasse. The terrorists were still demanding the release of over 700 Shiite prisoners in Israeli hands but Israel, like many other western nations, had a policy of not bowing to the demands of terrorists. It was, on the surface, a deadlock. Curiously enough the Israelis had been planning to release the prisoners in question before the hijack but could not now be seen to be doing so at the hijackers behest. The hijack had actually delayed their release rather than achieve it!

Late in the evening of Saturday June 15, the second full day of the hijack, it became apparent that the hijackers were not planning to fly anywhere that day. The crew took the opportunity of trying to get some much needed sleep; they did not know when their next chance would come. Sleeping was not easy with the constant coming and going of negotiators and hijackers and, at 1.45am on the Sunday morning, the release of three more hostages. The hijackers ended the day by renewing their demands with the added threat that, if they were not obeyed by Sunday morning, they would fly to an unspecified destination and destroy the aircraft killing the remaining passengers at the same time.

Sunday dawned and the captive Shiites had not been released. Captain Testrake was ordered to take the aircraft, once again, back to Beirut. With immense fatigue engulfing him and his crew, the only saving grace was that the route was now becoming familiar to him!

Flight 847 being an American aircraft with American citizens on board, President Reagan had been considering all the options with his advisers. Military intervention was one such option but, mindful of the daring attack of the Air France A300 at Entebbe airport by a crack team of Israeli commandos which killed all the hijackers but also cost the lives of many of the rescue team and one passenger, such an action was ruled out.

Another factor was that the permission to land in Algeria had been granted on the basis that there would be no violence whilst the aircraft was there. Reagan had to honour that promise to the Algerian leader. They decided that it was best to allow the hijack to run its course and to play each move as the occasion demanded. Nonetheless the mighty US Sixth Fleet was moved nearer the scene and put on radio silence in case the situation became intractable.

On the ground once more in Beirut the hijackers called for food and newspapers, they were obviously vain as well as brutal; they wanted to see what reaction their terrorism was having on the rest of the world. Later in the day they called for a meeting with Nabih Berri, the leader of the Amal group, with representatives of the Red Cross and with the ambassadors of Britain, France and Spain. Realising that the Red Cross was probably the most influential organisation in the drama, they urged them to resolve the matter quickly. The message didn't say it, but it seemed to read between the lines 'So we can all go home'!

Were the hijackers tiring and was their resolve fading? Their communique ended ominously stating that their next communique would be their last. What did that mean? The negotiators had to work it out, there were no further clues.

A meeting did take place a Nabih Berri's Beirut residence where Berri acted as the representative for the hijackers. Berri, head of the Amal militia, was known as a moderate amongst the fanatical groups and much rested on his negotiating skills. Early Monday morning the remaining passengers were removed from the aircraft and taken to another secret location in Beirut. There were now at least three groups of hostages in different and secret locations in Beirut but it was impossible to determine exactly where they were or how many were in each group.

The crew continued to be held on board the aircraft, they did not know why but assumed that the hijackers may still have plans for the aircraft if their demands were not met, plans that might well be a suicide flight. The prospects were very grim. Captain Testrake continued his efforts to support his crew and give them hope but he was continually frustrated by the refusal of the hijackers to give him free access the crew members in the cabin.

At one stage the hijackers displayed some humanity when they allowed an ambulance to be brought to the aircraft to take a sick male passenger off to hospital. It seemed that the additions to the hijack team during the Algiers stopover were less aggressive than the two original terrorists and that they might now be attempting to redeem their international image with some kind gestures.

Wednesday morning came, the sixth day of captivity for the crew on the aircraft and passengers still held in Beirut. The hijackers made an extraordinary decision. They invited the press to meet the still guarded flight crew at the aircraft. Representatives of Agence France and ABC News walked across the tarmac to see Captain Testrake leaning out of the cockpit window with the ominous hooded figure of an armed hijacker in the background.

They were allowed to talk to all three crewmembers in turn. Captain Testrake, unshaven but cheerful in the circumstances, cautioned against armed intervention saying it would result in their death since they were constantly under armed guard. Flight Engineer Benjamin Zimmerman, who was also a Lutheran pastor, said that the crew had prayed for their release and Testrake commented that "The Lord has seen us through trying times and He will see us through to the end". The prayers had worked thus far!

The interview came to an abrupt end when the driver of a food van who doubled as press photographer, pretending to know one of the hijackers, approached the aircraft. His camera was spotted by one of the gunmen who shot at him with his AK 47 and then sprayed bullets over the heads of the other newsmen. They packed their notepads and retreated!

Later in the day the gunmen requested toiletries and toothbrushes for the flightcrew who were urgently in need of a good freshen up. Food continued to be sent to the aircraft at regular intervals and Captain Testrake had commented as he talked to the press that "On the whole, the food's OK."

Apart from the flightcrew, the aircraft hijack was now effectively over leaving the negotiators to deal with the question of the hostages now held somewhere in Beirut. Captain Testrake, First Officer Phillip Maresca and Engineer Officer Benjamin Zimmerman, all of whom were still confined to the aircraft, had done their job and done it well, as had the crew in the cabin. They had contained the hijack with the exception of one tragic murder, now the wheels of politics and diplomacy had to grind their way to a face saving solution for all.

While negotiations took place on the world stage, the situation in Beirut descended into a farce. The Amal authorities arranged a series of press interviews. One interview featured the captives holding the weapons, not the captors, and everyone in a very relaxed mood. There was little doubt that it was a carefully planned public relations exercise probably directed by various Arab leaders to minimise the harm done so far. There is also no doubt that some passengers were demonstrating clear signs of the Stockholm Syndrome, a psychological condition when a captive will bond with the captor and even defend them against criticism. The spokesman for the group was eventually replaced by the passengers as being far too friendly with their former tormentors.

The following Wednesday, June 26, twelve days after the hijack commenced, Nabih Berri held a press conference in the basement of his office, obviously it was under the pressure of threats of unknown action by the United States if the matter was not resolved quickly. He announced the release of a male passenger with a heart condition on humanitarian grounds and then, out of the blue and almost as a casual aside he said "We are prepared to hand the kidnapped persons over to a Western embassy, Swiss or French whichever they choose." "Or," he added, "We can send the aeroplane to Damascus with the hostages."

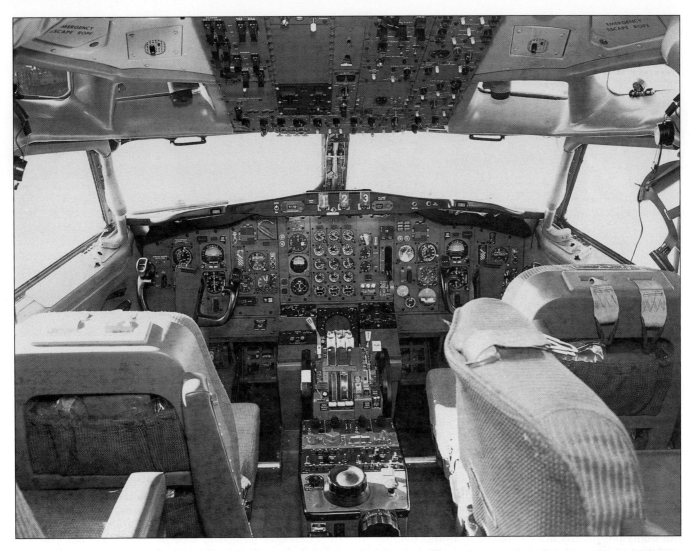

Cockpit of the 727 accommodating the captain (left seat), first officer (right seat) and the flight engineer who operates from a side mounted panel behind both pilots. (Boeing)

This was conditional that the hostages would not be finally released to go home until all Shiite prisoners held by the Israelis were freed. The impasse had been broken and President Assad, who had been in contact with the US President and offering to assist, agreed that the remaining hostages could all be taken to Damascus. They would not travel on the TWA 727 though; it was now well overdue for some regular servicing.

The following Saturday the hostages were assembled in a schoolyard near the airport ready for the start of their repatriation, however, the flightcrew and four passengers were missing. The following day they were finally joined by the missing flightcrew and passengers and together transported to Damascus by road. It was an impressive cavalcade with armed guards from the Amal and Druze militia, Red Cross representatives and Syrian army officers and security agents. All were headed by a Lebanese army truck mounted with an anti-aircraft gun! As they commenced the uncomfortable journey of just under four hours, they were presented with gifts and flowers by their captors. Reporters were kept well at bay. Grenades were rolled towards them and bursts of gunfire were aimed over their heads whenever they came too close to the convoy for the liking of those in charge.

At Damascus airport a C-141 US Air Force Starlifter was waiting to fly the hostages to Frankfurt to connect with a TWA flight back to the US. On July 1 they touched down on American soil at Andrews Air Force Base to be met by President and Mrs Reagan who boarded the aircraft and spoke with them all. America was about to celebrate Independence Day, July 4th. With their freedom restored it seemed a very appropriate time to come home.

Handling the hijack situation takes great tact and no little courage. It definitely pays to keep a low profile and to play along with the demands until outside agencies can resolve the crisis.

Captain Testrake and his crew had followed those principles well and if this account seems to down play the part the crew played in the successful outcome, it is simply because they were deliberately 'down playing' their role as the actual crewmembers throughout. There is little doubt though that the endurance, fortitude and bravery of Captain Testrake and all his crew had significantly contributed to the eventual successful outcome of a terrifying act of piracy in the air.

Efficient security measures are obviously vital to the travellers' wellbeing as this account clearly demonstrates and whilst in place at most of the world's

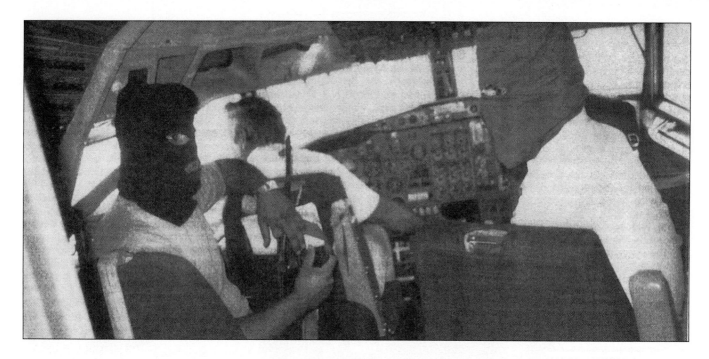

The hijackers in the cockpit with Captain Testrake. (Gamma-Liason)

airports, they are not always carried out proficiently. Many carriers, fed up with constant security breaches at Athens airport and elsewhere have established their own security checks manned by their own selected and well trained staff. Today not only is your hand baggage scrutinised, machines called 'sniffers' check the hold-stowed baggage and cargo is closely monitored. A worldwide system of intelligence has been established to enable airlines to increase security levels as required. It is hard to totally prevent hijacking but many improvements emanated from this event.

What can the individual do to improve travel safety? Simply fly with airlines with a good record and reputation for efficiency and avoid known areas of terrorism if you can. Lastly, security staff do not take kindly to flippant remarks when they ask the necessary questions concerning the packing and contents of your bags. Many an innocent passenger has been offloaded for such imprudence. The price of safety is eternal vigilance – you too can help.

Postscript – *The events of September 11th in New York and Washington DC have opened a new chapter in air terrorism. Obviously the security precautions in place were not adequate for this unexpected and totally new level of violence and for the heightened levels of planning and expertise by those bent on destruction and mayhem. The result will be further and more stringent security measures and increased cost to the traveller. Check-in procedures will become ever more complex as the security is heightened and it is likely that measures such as little or no carry on baggage, as well as a ban on outbound duty free may be introduced.*

Passenger profiling will be the norm, not just for when high risk security levels are put in place. There is little doubt that the airline intelligence networks are already being enhanced which will mean that from time to time a perfectly innocent traveller will be inadvertently under scrutiny and subject to questioning as the finer filter on the security net catches the minnows as well as the sharks. All of this will be intrusive into personal freedoms but essential while this madness is abroad. It will require understanding from the travelling public and enhanced diplomacy from airline staff as passengers are put through the vital security mill.

CHAPTER SEVEN

The Gimli Glider

RECIPE FOR DISASTER – Ingredients

Metric conversion
Mixed fleet using metric and Imperial data
Minor fuel sensor defect
Fuel gauges out of action
Helpful mechanic
Confusing documentation
Inadequate procedures
False but familiar premises

Mix all ingredients well, leave to mature for a few hours and dispatch aircraft.

When a commercial aircraft has an accident or serious incident, for years it has been the undesirable custom of the airline or authorities, when the cause is complex or not readily provable, to put the cause down the pilot error.

The Air New Zealand Mount Erebus disaster was one such example. In that case though, subsequent enquiries completely exonerated the crew from blame and determined that it was other factors that had set in train the series of events that caused the tragic crash.

This was also the case when an Air Canada Boeing 767 ran out of fuel midflight. Happily this aircraft, Air Canada Flight 143 with its passengers and cargo, was brought safely back to earth by the extraordinary skill and courage of Captain Bob Pearson, First Officer Maurice Quintal and their crew.

To land 'deadstick' on a runway, assuming there is a runway within reach, requires a lot of luck and an enormous amount of skill, it is not an emergency that can be adequately practised in the simulator.

With all the safety checks and crosschecks, the sophistication of modern jet airliners, the intense training which the crew undergo and regular checks of their skills, what could place a scheduled airline flight at 41,000 feet in cruise, many miles from its destination with no fuel remaining?

The sequence of events started some four years before the flight took place!

In 1979 Canada 'went metric' in common with the growing international trend. The old Imperial measurements of gallons (already complicated by the American gallon being different from the English gallon) and pounds were replaced by litres and kilograms although the aircraft speed continued to be measured in knots (nautical miles per hour) and its height determined in feet in accordance with international practice.

As with the conversion in other countries there was an intense period of public education but many citizens had trouble coming to grips with the new concept and had deep-rooted memories of all the old yardsticks. When police said they were looking for a suspect 1.85m tall most Canadians found it difficult to envisage how

tall that was but if they had been told that the suspect was just over six foot they could immediately picture that height.

Air Canada's fleet still had the instrumentation for the old Imperial measures and so fuel, oil etc continued to be ordered and measured in the old measurements. Add to that the fact that fuel required for a flight for commercial jet aircraft is ordered by weight which is then converted into a volume (gallons or litres) for measurement by the tanker delivering the fuel. The crews and ground handlers had carried out all of these conversions on a daily basis with perfect safety. But then entered the next ingredient for the dramatic incident yet to come.

A new fleet of Boeing 767s had been ordered by Air Canada and these came equipped to record the fuel and oil requirements and usage in litres & kilograms so now Air Canada had a fleet, most of which used Imperial measurements but with the new aircraft using the metric system. A recipe for disaster as it later proved.

The Boeing 767 which was to feature shortly had had an ongoing and intermittent minor defect, one of those that is hard to nail down. The electronic messages from the fuel processors that recorded the fuel on board in each tank and how much had been used were not getting through to the fuel gauges in the cockpit.

There were two channels to each fuel processor and the second channel was designed to automatically take over should the primary channel fail. As an added safety design feature each channel operated from a different power source – the system appeared foolproof. An intermittent electrical problem though was allowing a small current through to one of the channels so that it apparently had not failed and the other channel did not therefore automatically cut in. This problem had repeatedly re-occurred on the Boeing 767 registered as 604.

A mechanic assigned to the problem had established that channel one was operating normally and by only resetting the circuit breaker (fuse) for channel one he could keep the troublesome number two channel out of the circuit. The system then worked normally supplying information to the cockpit fuel gauges.

A check of the 'Minimum Equipment List' (MELs), the bible of what equipment the aircraft could and could not depart without, revealed that it was legal to allow the aircraft to operate with only one channel of the fuel processor working pending a spare part becoming available. There was an overriding proviso that the fuel quantity had to be manually checked by dripping the tanks at each stop.

'Dripping' the tanks is a simple procedure, which had been in use for years and found to be thoroughly reliable. A hollow tube, which extends into each fuel tank, is drawn down from under the wing. When fuel drips from the tube the top end has come down to the level of the surface of the fuel so the level of the fuel in the tank is known. The calibration is read from the 'dripstick' and applied to a set of tables which correct for wind incidence and any slope on the hardstanding. This provides the exact amount of fuel remaining in the tank.

The technician detailed to carry out the drip and dispatch the aircraft read the maintenance log and noted the fact that the circuit breaker for number two channel had been locked out and that the fuel gauges were functioning normally. Curious as to why this was so when the other channel was designed to take over automatically and having a few moments on his hands, he decided to do another check on the system. To do this he temporarily reset the number two channel circuit breaker, clearly labelled 'inop' (inoperative) with a yellow warning tape, intending to pull the circuit breaker again after the test. Unknown to him, this immediately caused all the fuel readouts to once again go blank.

With fatal inevitability there was a sudden press of service personnel in the cockpit carrying out routine tasks and he was reminded by a colleague that time was running short and he still had the drips to do. He forgot to once again pull the number two channel circuit breaker.

Proceeding with dripping the tanks he established that there were 7682 litres of fuel already on board. That would have to be made up to the Captain's fuel order of 22,300 kilograms, sufficient for the aircraft to transit Ottawa and fly on to Edmonton without refuelling. It was a simple task, he merely had to convert the existing litres to kilograms, determine the kilograms of extra fuel required and then, since the tanker measured its delivery in litres, convert his figure back to litres for the fuel order. These calculations were a daily routine for ground staff but, for whatever reason, he began to get a mental block.

The crew had now boarded the aircraft and First Officer Maurice Quintal noticed that the mechanic was having trouble with his figures and offered to help and, seeing the refueller at the back of the cockpit waiting for the fuel order, asked him for the specific gravity of the fuel (its weight per litre). The fueller, unaware that they needed to convert litres to kilograms and being totally unfamiliar with the complexities of the aircraft operation, provided the figure for litres to pounds which was over twice the correct figure. Thus when the calculations were complete the crew were ordering less than half the fuel by weight that they needed for the flight.

Captain Bob Pearson entered the cockpit. A 26 year veteran with Air Canada and highly experienced, as a matter of routine he checked the maintenance log. Seeing an item referring to the manual containing the MELs concerning the fuel sensors he looked it up to satisfy himself that everything was satisfactory.

"One may be inoperative provided fuel loading is confirmed by use of a measuring stick or by tender uplift after each fuelling and FMC fuel quantity information is available"

Having confidence in the foolproof drip system and that the defect had been checked out by qualified company technicians and rectification deferred in accordance with company manuals, he commenced his pre-flight procedures. His commendable caution though prompted him to double check this all with an Air Canada maintenance engineer who visited the flight deck. He was assured that the aircraft had been cleared by the company Maintenance Control Section pending replacement of the faulty fuel sensor.

The third pilot, who had acted as flight engineer was no longer carried on the latest 'glass cockpit' fully computerised Boeing 767s. This aircraft was designed to be operated by only two pilots and although aircrew associations had fought the removal of the flight engineer from the crew, it had been a losing battle.

The flight engineer, or the third pilot acting as flight engineer, had been responsible for all fuel calculations and was practised in that area. Now that responsibility was becoming unclear; there were no definitive rules as to whose duty it was to carry out this vital task. Adding to the confusion was the fact that the figure suggested by the fueller for the conversion of litres to the fuel weight was in use and correct for the rest of Air Canada's fleet of aircraft. The new Boeing 767 being the only aircraft using kilograms for fuel weight.

Departure time was looming and, as with all departures, the activity level was increasing but the Captain still wanted a further check that the correct fuel was on board for the flight through Ottawa and on to Edmonton. The fueller was not aware of this plan and was confident that the fuel loaded was very adequate for a flight to Ottawa where he understood they would refuel as normal. He refuelled this service frequently and was familiar with the usual fuel required.

The Captain was presented with the load sheet which he carefully checked, but he was presented with the false premise of the incorrect conversion figure and, like the others, being a familiar figure, he did not pick up the fact that the fuel volume had been converted to pounds not kilograms. He did note that the fuel was very slightly down on his order so he requested a 'top up' to the correct order. This caused another slight delay whilst the tanker returned and was reconnected. The extra fuel was loaded and the ground staff carried out yet another drip still unaware that the Captain planned to transit Ottawa without refuelling. They were happy with the fuel on board.

The scene was now set. The calculations had been checked by several people, the fuellers were happy, the maintenance control had cleared the aircraft for flight with the defective gauges and certified it as airworthy in the logbook in accordance with the MELs. Despite lingering unease there appeared to be no reason to further delay the aircraft without a 'please explain' from the management.

With the system failure, the departure fuel figure had to be manually loaded into the Flight Management Computer (FMC). From that time the computer would accurately record the fuel usage and calculate the fuel remaining throughout the flight but the figure loaded into the FMC was for the pounds of fuel – not the kilogram figure ordered!

The flight to Ottawa was uneventful except for a momentary recurrence of the bleed air valve problem, which was noted, and a maintenance check was requested on the company radio when they made their

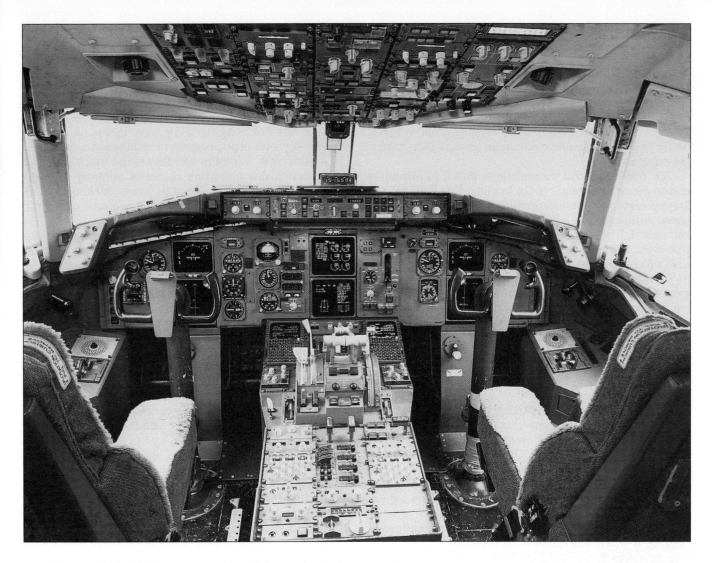

Cockpit of the Boeing 767. Note the flat panel displays replacing the array of 'steam gauges' of older design flightdecks. Mixed with a variety of means in which to measure the crucial jetfuel load pumped aboard the aircraft, human error ultimately led to a critical situation only saved by human skill in piloting the powerless aircraft to a deadstick landing. (Boeing)

inbound call. As an extra precaution, and needing to know how much fuel remained for the ongoing flight to Edmonton, the Captain also requested another fuel drip prior to his departure. The FMC would lose power on engine shut down in Ottawa and no longer record the fuel used from the initial entry in Montreal.

On arrival, Captain Pearson was discussing the bleed air valve problem with the mechanics and was making arrangements for departure should the problem recur on start up when the fueller arrived with the drip figures and reported the litres remaining in the tanks. The Captain requested the specific gravity of the fuel the fueller replying "1.78". Not knowing the Captain needed kilograms not pounds, the fueller had provided the figure giving the weight in pounds per litre of fuel.

Travelling on the flightdeck that day was an Air Canada maintenance expert Rick Dion. Hearing the specific gravity figure provided to the Captain, he was surprised. He recollected from his days in the Royal Canadian Air Force a figure of around .8 kilo per litre but assumed this unfamiliar figure had something to do with the recent metric changeover. He said nothing; another safety stop had passed by.

The Captain converted the litre figures using the specific gravity figure given which gelled with the figure

used out of Montreal and found that he had more than sufficient fuel for the flight on to Edmonton. Now, with the fuel load confirmed and a check of the bleed air valve arranged, they were ready to start up and depart for their final destination. The die was cast.

Full power was used for takeoff and the aircraft climbed very fast. This was probably the last clue to the impending disaster but there was no reason to believe that the aircraft was considerably lighter than planned. The extra climb rate could have simply been due to a slight wind shear.

They reached their cruising altitude of Flight Level 390 (39,000 feet) but, being more economical to cruise at a higher level, Captain Pearson requested a climb to Flight Level 410 and a clearance direct to Edmonton under radar. The flight proceeded normally with the crew completing the deck log with the time and fuel remaining over the various checkpoints. With the direct clearance and higher altitude they had made up fuel and time, everything was looking rosy.

Suddenly the warning light for the forward wing tank fuel pump illuminated indicating low pressure or failure. Simultaneously a written message appeared on the EICAS (Engine Indication and Crew Alerting System) screen spelling out the problem. A single fuel pump failure was not a great problem, there are two pumps in each tank and the fuel will gravity feed at most power settings.

Almost immediately another EICAS message informed them that the aft pump was also failing. This was still not a major emergency but, for safety's sake, Captain Pearson requested a clearance direct to Winnipeg, the nearest approved company alternate aerodrome. Far better to sort this problem out on the ground than have it get nasty in the air.

Air Traffic Control cleared them direct to Winnipeg and to descend as required for landing. The FMC (Flight Management Computer) provided them with their descent profile for the northwesterly runway at Winnipeg, runway 31. The FMC, preprogrammed by hand, showed that they had 11,000 kilograms of fuel remaining, just under four hours endurance.

Uncertain of the exact nature of the problem they switched on the more powerful fuel pumps in the centre wing tank to access any residual fuel and to give greater pressure to the fuel feeding the engines. They had only descended a few thousand feet when the failure lights for all six fuel pumps illuminated simultaneously. It was simply not feasible for all six pumps to fail at once; they had to assume it was low pressure due to fuel starvation, the worst possible scenario.

Captain Pearson needed to let his Flight Service Director, Bob Desjardins, know that there could be a developing problem. Rick Dion went back and told Bob to report to the Captain adding, "He has a problem".

Bob Desjardins entered the flightdeck and was told that they were diverting to Winnipeg with a fuel problem and would arrive in about 20 minutes. Not knowing exactly what the problem was the Captain also ordered Desjardins to brief the cabin crew for an emergency landing, it was always safer to be prepared for the worst case scenario.

As the crew were informed and gathered for a briefing the awful realisation came to them that all the lectures in the safety procedures school might now become reality and the mental shock left some of them concerned. Meanwhile the F/O called Air Canada Winnipeg on the company radio and briefed them on the problem. The engines were still running however, but not for long.

The first to fail was the left engine. The shutdown checklist was completed. Captain Pearson declared a full emergency, not for the single engine failure but for the fact that the combination of circumstances and that the exact reason for the failure was not known.

With a single engine failure the checklist called for a landing at the nearest suitable airport, this seemed a little different. He informed the controllers that he now required the southerly runway which would require less time and manoeuvring for his approach and landing. The weather was fine and with only light winds fortunately either runway was suitable.

Without warning the second engine failed and, with it, an almost total power failure in the cockpit. They broadcast a Mayday and requested radar direction to any airfield within range.

With both engines failed and not driving the generators they only had a limited life battery to supply bare essentials. The checklist called for them to start the Auxiliary Power Unit, a small jet in the tail, which could provide some electrical power but they had no success.

The dreadful reality hit them; they were totally out of fuel, in clouds with limited flying instruments.

Captain Pearson ordered the Ram Air Turbine to be deployed which gave them some hydraulic power for the flying controls but they would have to use the emergency systems to extend the landing gear and flaps and with the electrical power gone even emergency flap extension was not possible. They were facing an extreme emergency with little prospect of a successful outcome.

A glide with a total power loss is not much different to a normal descent when power is minimal with the engines just idling. The trouble comes making the approach when there is practically no control over both height and speed at the same time.

To land 'deadstick' on a runway, assuming there is a runway within reach, requires a lot of luck and an enormous amount of skill, it is not an emergency that can be adequately practised in the simulator. Captain Pearson set the aircraft on its best glidespeed to extract maximum distance but he had no instruments to tell him his rate of descent so he could not tell how far he could take the aircraft in a glide. He could time his altitude change against the clock but the workload was high enough already.

He would have to rely on the controller to provide such information but now with the loss of electrical power, the transponder was not providing height and other data on the controller's radar screen, just the primary 'blip'. He could no longer help them assess how far they could glide to possible safety.

The problems confronting Captain Pearson on landing were many and varied. He would have to exhibit supreme judgement to avoid landing short or running off the far end of any runway at high speed. He had no knowledge of how fast the landing gear would extend in the circumstances and whether he would have any flaps to provide drag and help slow the aircraft for a safe landing. It would all be 'seat of the pants' flying with perhaps sideslipping to lose height and possibly a wheels up or partial gear landing. There were too many unknown factors to be able to make any plans, he had to take it as he found it and play it 'off the cuff'.

The controller advised them that they were 65 miles from Winnipeg and 45 miles from Gimli field, not a major airport but F/O Quintal recollected that it had a good long runway and it was closer. Better a bird in the hand and Winnipeg was starting to look uncomfortably distant. The controller requested the vital information for a major emergency, souls on board and fuel remaining!

They had closed to less than 40 miles from Winnipeg. F/O Quintal had run up a descent profile on his notepad and he didn't like what he saw. He crosschecked the figures and realised that, whilst the weather was favourable, it was simply too far away, they would be landing around 12 miles short of the airport on unknown ground. Gimli too was looking marginal but it was closer.

Suddenly, through a break in the cloud they spotted an airfield just ahead.

"What's the airfield ahead of us now?" Captain Pearson tersely asked the controller.

He was informed that it was a disused airfield called Netley and its condition was unknown – not a good prospect perhaps. The controller had been frantically doing his own calculations and he too believed that Flight 143 would not be able to glide to Winnipeg. There had to be a change of plan, Gimli now looked like the only choice.

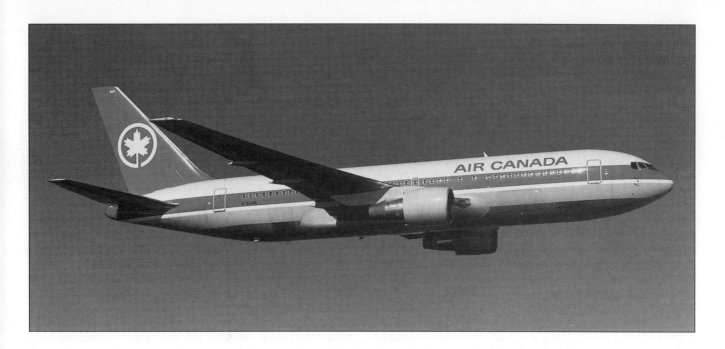

A Boeing 767-200 of Air Canada. (Boeing)

Gimli had been a RCAF base operating the early, relatively low powered jet fighters, Shooting Stars or T-33s, as they were known. As a consequence it had highly desirable long twin runways. Closed as a RCAF base long ago, it was now used on occasions by the Winnipeg Car Club who ironically were having a meeting that day. Fortunately lady luck started to smile on Flight 143 for the car meet was over and the enthusiasts were returning to their parking area.

Winnipeg ATC quickly managed to track down some details of Gimli airfield and passed them to the stricken aircraft. They had also, in an incredibly short space of time available, to locate and dispatch emergency vehicles to Gimli. The Winnipeg fire crews and ambulances simply could not get there in time, besides they had to stay on duty at the operating airport as the law required. Two nearby military bases were contacted and asked to scramble ambulances, fire vehicles and helicopters with supplies and first aid crews.

Winnipeg then contacted a small airport nearby and got them to broadcast an alert on 'guard' frequency telling all aircraft to keep well clear of Gimli, the Winnipeg controller's radio transmissions would not reach low flying aircraft that far away. Another Air Canada aircraft in cruise also broadcast the alert, Flight 143 had to be able to manoeuvre freely, as best it could, and did not need the extra problem of avoiding other aircraft.

In the cabin, the crew had now been fully briefed and, in turn, had briefed the passengers for a full emergency landing. Such a briefing, understandably, always arouses great fear in passengers who are unable to do anything but sit there and place their trust in the skills of the pilots and crew.

There was a lot of reassuring to be done in addition to the safety briefing. Able bodied men were moved to emergency exits so they could be first out and assist other passengers away from the escape slides, others seated near exits, were briefed how to open them in the event that crew members were incapacitated. The cabin was now ready for the worst with the crew doing their best to show an air of confidence and calm at the same time concealing their own fears.

Flying any aircraft 'deadstick' requires a high degree of airmanship. Add to that all the uncertainties of this arrival and the fact that this was a Boeing 767, not a small recreational aircraft, and the prospects for a good outcome were not good, they would also need a good measure of luck.

They were now close to Gimli and clear of the cloud. Captain Pearson could see the approach lights and was flying visually with no further aid from the Air Traffic Controllers. He was lining up on the longer of the two runways on a northwesterly heading but it was this runway, due to its greater length, which was used as a drag strip by the motor enthusiasts. The Ram Air Turbine was providing power to the flying controls but he could not operate the landing flaps. He would have to touchdown at a much higher speed than normal for a flapless landing. Having no reverse thrust to slow the aircraft and only the emergency braking system available he knew that the high landing speed would almost certainly blow out his tyres on the rollout.

Captain Pearson tried to get information on the runway condition from Winnipeg but they were not able to help much, they had no reason to have up to date information on a disused airfield.

"Will there be anyone on the runway?" he enquired.

"We cannot tell you for sure," was the not so reassuring reply.

As they got closer it was apparent to the F/O that they were approaching much too fast and much too high. Better than landing short perhaps but undesirable nonetheless. The Captain considered making one orbit but that presented the danger of possibly losing too much height and he would lose sight of the runway and might not be correctly lined up with the runway as he came out of the turn. It was not an option. Their only choice was to lower the landing gear early but, once down it could not be retracted again, it could cause more drag than they needed – they were in uncharted territory.

The F/O selected the landing gear down on the Captain's order and they waited for the normal 'clunks' of the gear lowering and locking into place. There was no sound. They looked at each other without speaking; they both knew what it meant. Apart from no drag to solve their height and speed problem, it would be a wheels up landing. Not a great drama compared to their current situation but very noisy and certainly not the best option.

The F/O reached for the alternate gear extension control which merely released the gear doors allowing the landing gear to fall under their own weight. The gear released and the comforting noises were there but there was no certainty yet that it would lock into position but they did have the extra drag they needed. Then to their relief, two green lights illuminated indicating that the main wheels were down and locked. The nose gear was not in place, probably because it was lighter and, lowering forwards, it was fighting the slipstream unaided by hydraulic power.

They were still too fast. There was only one thing left, a last minute sideslip. They had sufficient speed to make it a safe manoeuvre. Sideslipping does increase the stalling speed of an aircraft and a stall at low level is certain death. After all the misfortunes leading up to the incident it was their extreme good fortune that day that Captain Pearson was an experienced glider pilot and very familiar with the correct technique.

The cabin crew, realising that a landing was imminent, ordered the passengers to brace, they didn't need an order to pray! The violent manoeuvre of the sideslip had told them all that things were far from normal. A light aircraft that had not heard the all-planes warning alert was waiting to line up on the right hand runway and the pilots suddenly saw this airliner in a violent, wing down, sideslip attitude on its final approach to the left runway. They thought they were about to witness at close quarters, a major aircraft catastrophe.

Captain Pearson bore the aircraft down towards the landing point unaware that his F/O, with a little more time to spare than he, had looked further ahead and seen people standing on the runway. He couldn't tell the Captain, there was no time. He could only hope that they would see the approaching aircraft and run for their lives. It was simply a question of a few peoples' lives at risk as opposed to the 65 plus souls on board the 767.

Captain Pearson held the sideslip as long as possible. Every knot of speed that he could lose prior to touchdown represented a lot shorter landing distance and the difference between leaving the far end of the runway at an undesirably high speed or maybe actually stopping within the confines of the runway. One of the people on the runway, a young boy, looked up, saw the aircraft about to touchdown, screamed a warning and ran for his life.

Flight 143 touched down 29 minutes after the emergency commenced, almost exactly what would be expected from a deadstick glide from 41,000 feet. Whilst landing fast due to the lack of landing flaps, the touchdown was in the correct landing area. There was sufficient runway to stop if all went well.

Then a huge noise as the nosewheel, by this time partially extended, folded back and the nose of the aircraft hit and scraped along the runway, a mixed blessing. Whilst uncomfortable and certainly terrifying for the passengers, in the absence of 'stopping power' from the reverse thrust systems, it would help.

The Captain looked down the runway and saw the fleeing boy and others who had been on the runway. He prepared to direct the aircraft off the runway to avoid them if he had to. He had no nose wheel steering and practically no rudder control. Then he saw a robust metal handrail set into the runway. If he hit that it could spear up through the fuselage and kill passengers. With a supreme effort he managed to slightly move the sliding aircraft to one side so that the rail ran down the side of the fuselage and not up and through it.

They finally came to the literal 'grinding halt' still on the runway. The two pilots completed the emergency shutdown procedures but now smoke was entering the flightdeck. This was coming from the red-hot fuselage under the nose where the nose wheel should have been. The magnesium content of the aircraft's skin can cause a very intense fire once it reaches a certain temperature; there was still danger.

An emergency evacuation was initiated in the cabin with cabin crew opening the doors and urging the passengers down the escape slides. The exaggerated nose-down attitude meant that the rear door slides, still useable, were just off the ground. It would be a wild ride down those but dangerous and incapacitating smoke was now entering the cabin. This gave that extra incentive to passengers to take the ride down the slides.

The motor club members who had been on the runway were now racing to the aircraft with any fire extinguishers they could find and they tackled the nose gear area where the smoke was worst. The Gimli fire brigade arrived very quickly and all traces of the fire were soon fully extinguished by them. The passengers were all safely able to safely leave the aircraft and gather at a safe distance for a headcount.

The success of this recovery from an impossible situation was such that, after minor repairs, the aircraft was ferried (crew only) to the company base at Winnipeg where the final extensive repairs brought it back to a full and safe operational condition.

Initially, Air Canada's enquiries put the cause of the accident down to pilot error and errors on the part of ground technicians and refuelling staff. There was a public outcry though and the government called for an independent enquiry which found that none of the above were to blame but that the causes were many and varied.

They found that having a fleet operating in both metric and Imperial measures was undesirable, that the company failed to clearly assign responsibilities for fuel calculations and that unclear, confusing and contradictory company manuals also played a part. The final finding of the chairman of the board of enquiry was that the professionalism and skill of the flightcrew and flight attendants overcame the corporate and equipment deficiencies and had avoided a major disaster.

Sometimes it takes a near accident of this severity and magnitude to make an airline take a closer look at their procedures and manuals. The review of all these factors undoubtedly increased the safety of civil aviation not only in that airline but also in the aviation industry in general. It certainly highlighted the dangers presented when multiple units of measurement were being used in the transition to 'metrification'.

CHAPTER EIGHT

Just a Minor Problem!

The best maintenance and quality control cannot always prevent a mechanical failure, as any motorist will attest. When your car breaks down you pull over and call for the road service company and possibly get towed home.

In the air it is a different matter, no pullover lanes there, the aircraft has to be brought back safely to land. In the following account of a midair 'breakdown' the skill of the captain and crew coupled with the captain's 'local knowledge' certainly saved the day.

The aircraft manufacturers had never envisaged their aircraft remaining in the air with such spectacular and severe damage. No preproduction tests could have simulated this failure, it was a totally unforeseen emergency and they were literally amazed that the crew had nursed the aircraft back for a safe landing.

On June 28 1965 Pan American World Airways Flight 843 was scheduled to operate the regular service across the North Pacific from San Francisco to Honolulu, a flight of around five hours. The Boeing 707-321B was under the command of Captain Charles H Kimes. Even at the relatively young age of 44 years he had accumulated over 17,700 flying hours experience. His First Officer Frederick Miller and Second Officer Max Webb were also very experienced and the Flight Engineer, Fitch Robertson had more hours than the Captain!

Through the huge orange fireball he could see that not only had the number four engine fallen off but also a large section of the outer wing was missing.

That day they had 143 passengers on board under the care of the two pursers and four stewardesses who made up the cabin crew. Most of the passengers were holiday makers bound for the tropical paradise of the Hawaiian Islands and many were travelling with their small children. They were not to arrive in Honolulu on this flight.

The takeoff run at San Francisco was routine; they lifted off and immediately selected the undercarriage up. The typical clunk and thump of the wheels locking into place and the gear doors closing was clearly heard in the passenger cabin and the aircraft continued its steep climbout to clear the hilly terrain surrounding the airport. They had only just climbed through 700 feet, well below the safety height for the area, when trouble struck.

The crew became aware of heavy vibration which was immediately identified as coming from number 4 engine, the Flight Engineer confirmed the source of the problem on his instrument panel and called,

"Engine failure number four."

Captain Kimes ordered the engine to be shut down and was just calling out the checklist actions when there was a violent shudder and instantaneously the number four engine fire warning switch illuminated accompanied by the fire warning bell. The clamour of the bell is designed to gain the crews' instant attention – it did that – but its noise is such that it can be a distraction to the subsequent emergency actions. First Officer Miller silenced the bell on the Captain's command and glanced back out of his window to see if there were visible signs of fire.

Although it was the outboard engine – hard to see on the severely swept back wing – he could easily see that this was not a false warning. A huge ball of fire was streaming from the area of number four engine and, from the black oily smoke that was trailing behind the aircraft, he knew that their jetfuel was feeding the fire. He thought that the outboard fuel tank had inexplicably exploded triggering the engine fire warning. He reported what he could see to the Captain.

S/O Max Webb could not see what was taking place from his position in the jump seat behind the Captain. If he left the seat he would have to pass in front of the Flight Engineer who needed free access to the centre console between the two pilots and, more importantly, to the thrust levers. Webb stayed in his seat and monitored all the actions and flying. He had the lowest workload of any of the crewmembers and would be a vital back up monitoring all the crews' actions and the aircraft's flightpath.

The First Officer had been flying up until the alarm sounded but company procedures called for the Captain to fly the aircraft in the event of an emergency. Captain Kimes took over the controls and, applying rudder to offset the yaw of the aircraft and setting maximum thrust on the other three engines to maintain their climb out, he now called the full engine fire checklist.

"Thrust lever close."

"Start lever cutoff."

"Engine Fire pull."

"Fire bottle discharge."

The First Officer meticulously identified the correct engine control for each item and indicated that he had carried out the action. He looked again at the wing and saw that the fire was not diminishing. As the engine fire checklist called for them to fire the second extinguisher bottle in one minute, he started the sweep second hand of the clock. Then, to his horror, the full extent of the emergency became evident.

Through the huge orange fireball he could see that not only had the number four engine fallen off but also a large section of the outer wing was missing. That accounted for the violent shudder and the noticeable wing drop as the fire warning had sounded. With it had gone the outboard aileron, a primary flying control, which limited their ability to keep the wings level and turn the aircraft. They had an unprecedented and potentially lethal emergency on their hands.

The First Officer's initial impression that a fuel tank had exploded was exactly correct but it was not the fuel tank that he had thought it was. The main outboard fuel tank (number 4 tank) was still in place, it was the empty reserve tank at the extremity of the wing (number 4 reserve) which had blown up, probably because it was empty for this short flight and contained only fuel air vapours – a deadly cocktail when the engine fire was raging so close to it. The explosion had weakened the outer wing structure and wreckage of the outer wing section was later found along a seven mile stretch of Flight 843's flightpath falling to earth as it disintegrated bit by bit.

The Captain urgently needed height for safe manoeuvring but as he did not want to further stress the severely damaged wing, he levelled off at one thousand three hundred feet, lower than the height for a normal circuit but safe enough once he was out over the sea. The aircraft now became very difficult to handle. The high power on the remaining three engines was yawing the aircraft to the right and was controllable, but the loss of lift from the right wing was adding considerably to his problems.

It was difficult enough to keep the aircraft straight and level, making necessary turns to return to an airfield would be a major battle. It took all the rudder trim and some good old fashioned leg muscle to keep directional control of his aircraft. He knew that the passengers would be well aware of the problem and, whilst still struggling to maintain control, was able to say a few calming words.

"Folks, as you can see we have a minor problem" he started off the announcement in his calm and languid American accent. The First Officer looked over to the Captain not believing what he was hearing and the Captain, seeing his questioning expression and realising what he had just said, quickly added,

"Well, I guess it's not so minor!"

The passengers had indeed seen the problem. All those on the right hand side of the aircraft had a clear view from the aircraft windows. The huge billowing orange flame streaming from the outer wing gradually turning into an oily black smoke trail behind the aircraft left many in no doubt that they were doomed. A small boy seeing the fire shouted out to his mother, other passengers heard and looked out too. Many prayed, there was little else they could do.

The Captain came on the public address once more with a further calming message. He wanted them to know that he had the visually appalling situation under control but nonetheless advised them to fit their life jackets and, most of all, to keep calm. A ditching off the coast was a very real probability at this stage. The cabin crew, working like the well trained team they were, needed no instructions from the Captain. They went about the cabin ensuring that all passengers had fitted their life jackets and briefing them for the emergency, be it a land or sea arrival. Their professional and calm demeanour did much to reassure the passengers and allay any possible panic.

US Coast Guard pilot Lieutenant Melvin Hartman had also seen the stricken 707 struggling to climb away. It was evident to him that it had incurred severe damage and that the spectacular fire, which he later said looked like a "Roman candle", was only one of the problems the pilot faced. He did not hesitate but immediately took off to fly wing on the 707 and provide whatever assistance he could.

Captain Kimes had sent out two Mayday calls but these were not heard by San Francisco controllers probably because the aircraft was so low that the transmissions were blocked by the hilly countryside surrounding the airport. Hartman began to relay all the calls from Flight 843; his presence was a great comfort to Captain Kimes who now knew that his every need could be quickly relayed to air traffic control.

As Flight 843 departed from San Francisco airport staff in the control tower had also seen the fire erupt from the starboard wing. They did not know exactly what the problem was or even how bad it was but they had immediately advised all inbound flights on their radio frequency to 'standby' and that there was an emergency in progress.

Fellow pilots now knew that one of their own was in trouble and would assist the controllers in their efforts to get the flight safely back to land. The San Francisco airport emergency vehicles were alerted and local hospitals were put on standby to receive patients if the worst eventuated.

PanAm pilots frequently practised 'engine out' procedures, it is part of the routine and ongoing training for all airline pilots, but nothing had prepared Captain Kimes or his crew for flying or landing with a large section of a wing missing. He had to make some quick decisions and they had to be right. Any false move or delay might aggravate the structural damage and set in train an uncontrolled plummet to the ground or sea with the inevitable results.

Whilst Captain Kimes had the aircraft under some semblance of control, the emergency was far from over. The emergency checklist actions had successfully extinguished the engine fire and it was probably good fortune that the blazing engine had fallen from the aircraft. Jetfuel was now streaming from broken feed lines and could have easily reignited had the blazing engine still been in place, broken electrical wires were flailing in the slipstream and could short out at anytime causing an unwanted spark. There was still the very real possibility that the fire could break out again.

The quickest possible landing was essential but that had to be tempered with landing at the most suitable airfield. He remembered that just to the north of San Francisco lay the massive Travis Air Force Base with a much longer runway than any at San Francisco. There were only three realistic alternative, Travis, San Francisco International or the ever present possibility that he might have to ditch in the ocean before the aircraft broke up.

In his mind he quickly went though the merits of the two possible airfields. On landing, there was always the possibility of the fire breaking out again. With the obviously damaged and leaking fuel lines, when the aircraft came to a stop on the runway there would be jetfuel everywhere. Having landed, there would be no slipstream to carry the fire away; burning fuel could engulf the aircraft as they came to a stop. They needed the very best in fire fighting equipment on hand; Travis not only

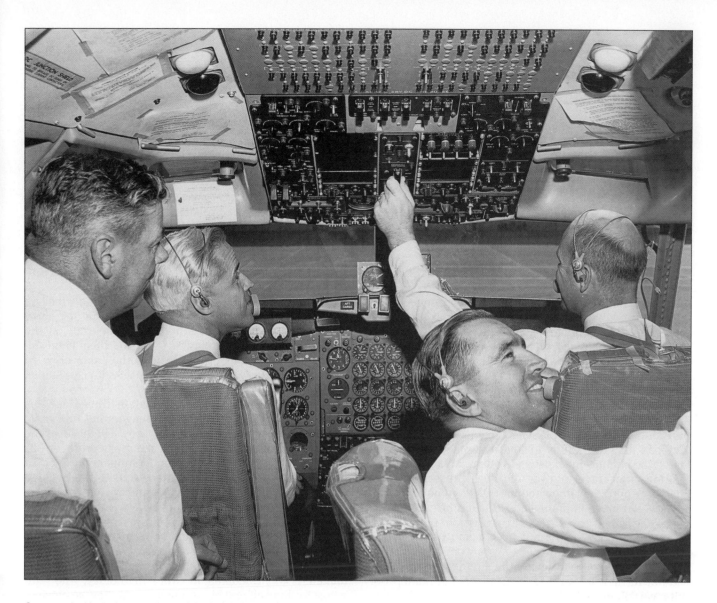

Compared with the later versions of the increasingly complex piston engined airliners of the 'fifties, the 707 jet was a relatively simple aircraft to fly and operate. Pictured is a 707 flightdeck of the period with the first officer and flight engineer performing checks under the watchful gaze of the captain (left front seat) and a Boeing observer prior to this aircraft's acceptance flight to the customer airline. (Boeing)

had that to handle the big military jets in an emergency but the base also had medical facilities on site. If there were injuries then they could be treated much sooner than if they landed back at San Francisco.

The question of control of the aircraft finally swayed him. With the loss of lift on the right side of the aircraft it was hard to turn to the left and, if he turned to the right it was an immense struggle to get the aircraft level again. Any turns had to be as gentle as possible as did his flying of the aircraft if they were to get down safely. Travis would be easier to get to so the decision was made to head for Travis and he informed air traffic control.

With Hartman still flying close by and relaying all his radio calls, he gently turned the aircraft towards the Air Force Base some 50 miles away. He was still very low having not dared to further stress the aircraft with a climb, at this altitude he was reliant on directions from the controllers for navigation and would not see his chosen destination until he was just a mile or so away. All the time the First Officer was keeping a constant check on the damaged right wing to alert the Captain if the situation worsened.

Once Captain Kimes had completed the turn to set course the relatively straight flight to Travis AFB gave him and the crew a brief respite. There were no major manoeuvres to carry out apart from small heading corrections, with the constant thrust setting he had been able to trim the aircraft and reduce the physical work required but soon it would all start again as they prepared for landing.

Just under 20 minutes after they had taken off on the ill fated flight they sighted the Travis AFB runway. The flight attendants had the cabin fully prepared for the emergency landing and for a rapid evacuation of the aircraft should it prove necessary. Preparing the aircraft for landing the Captain ordered,

"Gear down, before landing checklist."

The First Officer pulled the gear lever out of its stowed detent and selected it to the down position. Nothing happened! The primary hydraulic system had, not surprisingly, failed. They could try and trouble shoot and still attempt to lower the gear hydraulically but time was running out. Quicker to go straight to the manual lowering cranks which were there under the cockpit

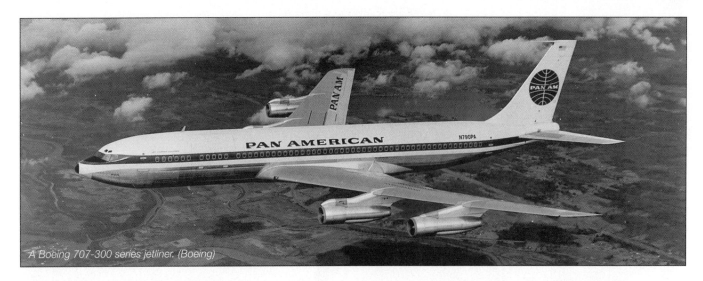
A Boeing 707-300 series jetliner. (Boeing)

floor. The first job was to descend to the cramped compartment under the cockpit and operate the nose gear release lever. This done, Second Officer Max Webb and the Flight Engineer returned to the cockpit to open the floor access hatches and rapidly crank the nose wheel gear down. They then set about tackling the cranks for each of the main undercarriage systems in turn. After several minutes of vigorous winding the gear fell into place and a quick check through the viewing windows in the floor of the main passenger cabin confirmed that they had all successfully locked into place. They completed the landing checklist and were ready to land.

Along the Travis runway the huge fire trucks were lined up where they expected the 707 to come to a stop. They would move in immediately the aircraft halted trying to extinguish any further fire or, at worst, control it. Their other vitally important task would be to ensure that escape routes for the passengers were kept clear of fire enabling them to evacuate the aircraft and run clear without further danger. Rescue personnel in flameproof suits were there too.

The aircraft touched down smoothly at 2.30pm exactly 20 minutes after they had lifted off for their flight to Honolulu, 20 minutes that neither the crew nor the passengers would ever forget.

The fire vehicles moved in quickly whilst ambulances and rescue vehicles held off at a safe distance. It soon became evident that the spilling jetfuel would not ignite as everyone had feared it might but as a precautionary measure the fire crews laid down extinguishing foam on the pooling jetfuel beneath the aircraft. The relieved passengers were able to make a safe and orderly disembarkation. Many wept as they walked away from the badly scarred aircraft; it was the relief of being once again on terra firma with a liberal dose of nervous reaction that caused the tears to flow. They had survived a seemingly impossible situation thanks to the skill of Captain Kimes and his crew and the rugged strength of the incredible Boeing 707 but it wasn't quite over yet!

Another PanAm aircraft was sent to Travis to pick up the long suffering passengers so that they could recommence their planned flight from San Francisco. As they waited and watched its arrival, before their very eyes the nose wheel collapsed and the aircraft skidded, nose on the runway, to an embarrassing halt! A third attempt with yet another aircraft was more successful.

Surprisingly, just barely recovered from their ordeal

and the grandstand view of the second aircraft's mishap on landing, they boarded the aircraft. During the short flight back, Captain Kimes addressed them all on the public address congratulating them for their calm demeanour that had made the task of the cabin crew so much easier. He was warmly and deservedly applauded by the grateful passengers.

Letters flooded in praising Captain Kimes and his crew, not only from admiring passengers but one came from Vice President Hubert Humphrey. The head of the Federal Aviation Agency Najeeb Halaby is on record as describing the brief flight as "A masterful feat of airmanship" and he duly presented Captain Kimes with a citation in recognition of his skills and tenacity.

The four cockpit crewmembers were also jointly presented with the Daedalian Award, presented annually to pilots or crews for great skill and airmanship in dealing with an emergency – a very appropriate award in view of the mythical character after whom the award was named. It was Daedalus, in Greek mythology, who built wings for himself and his son Icarus who flew so close to the sun that his wings melted!

Through it all Captain Kimes modestly maintained that it was the whole crew which had brought the flight home, not just himself or the cockpit crew alone, and that is true, but they had a fine leader.

Boeing had never contemplated preproduction testing for a partial wing loss. The explosive failure of the engine of Flight 843 at takeoff power had sent shards of steel through the compressors which were still rotating at high speed. The compressors had in turn disintegrated and torn open the plenum chambers which normally contained the searing heat of combustion in the engine.

The flame had torched out igniting fuel leaking from severed fuel lines and seared the wing itself. The combined damage caused by the catastrophic engine failure, the explosion of number four reserve fuel tank and the fire had weakened the wing structure which finally failed removing 25 feet of the surface that kept them in the air.

Boeing engineering experts were dumbfounded that the aircraft stayed in the air, let alone could still be controlled with around one third of the total span of one wing missing.

The incident clearly demonstrated the rugged reliability of the Boeing 707 under the most unusual circumstances and the prudence of the fail safe policy of the US aircraft construction industry and regulatory authorities.

CHAPTER NINE

"Uncontrol, Uncontrol – JL123"

In addition to the detailed investigations into major incidents and crashes, the conditions experienced by the crew are often recreated in a simulator to provide further clues as to what went wrong or how the crew contained, or failed to contain the situation.

The modern simulator, once inside, is a very realistic replica of the aircraft cockpit. From the outside it is just a huge box sitting on hydraulic jacks. Highly computerised, any emergency the aircraft may encounter can be simulated in perfect safety. All the movements of a real time flight can be reproduced so that pilots in the simulator get the same 'seat of the pants' input of what an aircraft would be doing.

Computer programs even permit training for flying into difficult airports with highly sophisticated projected images of the airport and surrounding terrain. At a cost of tens of millions of dollars each, they are expensive but considerably less expensive than using an aircraft for crew training.

One of the greatest values of the simulator for training is that it can be 'frozen' and the instructor can explain a procedure or, where the pilot was not flying to standard, the exercise can be repeated at little cost. I used this 'freeze' facility when I attempted to simulate the awful circumstances in which a Japan Airlines crew found themselves one day. After just a few minutes, far shorter than their ordeal, I had had enough. I was unable to realistically keep the aircraft flying and was physically drained. My admiration for their efforts could not be greater.

This is the one true story in this book, which does not have a happy ending, but it is a tale of superlative airmanship and courage and deserves a place.

The Boeing 747 was basically designed for long range intercontinental flying but due to the need for a large passenger capacity aircraft for the huge domestic market, Japan Airlines ordered the specially developed short range 747. It could carry 500 passengers in high density seating, quite acceptable for the short, inter island trips. The wings and undercarriage were considerably strengthened to take the wear and tear of the more frequent takeoffs and landings encountered in 'short haul' operations. It was called the Boeing 747SR of which Japan Airlines had nine aircraft in their fleet.

After completing four flights of mostly business commuters on August 12th 1985 this aircraft, registered JA8119, was scheduled to operate from Tokyo's Haneda Airport to Osaka, a short flight of under one hour when they would not even reach the normal higher cruising levels. Two new pilots joined for the flight, Captain Takahama, a senior training captain was in command and conducting promotional training for a 747 First Officer. Captain Takahama had served 19 years with Japan Air where he had accumulated over 12,500 hours of experience. He occupied the instructional right hand seat with his command trainee sitting in the left hand command seat under his supervision.

This evening flight was mostly full of families making the traditional return to their birthplace for the three day Japanese festival of Bon, a time when ancestors are remembered. Unusually for the extremely busy Haneda airport, this flight, Japan Air 123 departed almost exactly on schedule with its 509 passengers and crew. At 6.12pm JL123 lifted off and set course down the airway system for Osaka climbing to their planned cruising level of 24,000ft (flight level 240).

Shortly after departure the crew requested 'track shortening' and obtained a direct clearance from the Tokyo radar controller, all flights in this high traffic density area being constantly monitored by radar.

So far it had been a routine flight, they had now reached their cruising level and the autopilot was locked in controlling the aircraft and navigating

The few moments of relatively good control of the aircraft were short lived and despite using the landing gear and discussing the use of flaps, the aircraft now had a mind of its own with little the crew could do to control height or direction. They were now below 9000 feet and heading towards the mountainous countryside in central Honshu.

it, under the watchful eyes of the pilots, to its destination. Suddenly, there was a total loss of cabin pressure. A terrifying loud bang came from the rear of the fuselage accompanied by the appearance of a white mist as moisture in the cabin air condensed out with the loss of pressure.

Vent holes in the cabin floor, designed to equalise pressure between the cabin and the cargo hold in just such an event, opened preventing greater damage to the structure. The passenger oxygen masks fell from the ceiling and the recorded announcement telling passengers to don the oxygen masks started broadcasting in the cabin, which was backed up by the public address announcement by cabin staff. The passengers and cabin crew were only too well aware that some serious emergency had occurred.

The crew on the flightdeck were also well aware of the problem, the cabin pressure warning horn was blaring and the pressure change was very evident on their eardrums. The Captain ordered the transponder to be switched to the emergency code and the crew set about carrying out the emergency procedures and determining the cause of the problem. They had been in cruise just one minute. On seeing the emergency transponder 'squawk' on his screen, the controller immediately cleared the aircraft to return to Haneda as they requested and gave them a radar heading to the Oshima radio beacon for their return.

Before the crew could carry out the drills for the decompression though the Captain realised that they were losing hydraulic pressure. All the controls are operated by hydraulic pressure and the four systems, one powered by each engine, are regarded as fail safe since any one system will still provide reduced control. The autopilot consequently also relies on hydraulic pressure for its correct operation.

The Flight Engineer monitored the rapidly diminishing loss of hydraulic fluid until, nine seconds after the cabin warning horn had started sounding, all hydraulic pressure was lost and with it, all normal control of the aircraft

The radar controller was keenly watching the 'paint' of JL123 on his radar screen. He had cleared them for a right turn of nearly 180° to the Oshima beacon to head the aircraft for home but was amazed to see it only turn about 50° and head off in the wrong direction to the northwest. He called and asked the aircraft the nature of their emergency but, not surprisingly, did not get a reply. The aircraft's height, shown on his radar screen, was varying considerably from the flight level they were supposed to be at. He repeated the clearance to turn onto 090° for the return to Oshima. Now the aircraft mysteriously replied,

"But now uncontrol."

The controller called for a discrete radar code on the transponder to assist in keeping the aircraft clearly identified on his screen but again there was no reply. He asked if the aircraft could descend and this time the crew replied that they were already descending. The controller, not yet knowing the nature of the emergency was unable to provide assistance that might be needed.

"Right – your position 72 miles to Nagoya. Can you land at Nagoya?" he enquired, attempting to offer them a nearer airport for landing.

"Negative – request back to Haneda" came the reply.

The controller was doing his best to give them what he saw as the safest course of action. The exchanges were in the international language of the air, English, and realising that something very serious had occurred giving the crew no time to inform him of the exact situation the controller suggested they continue in Japanese, which would certainly help the beleaguered crew.

The aircraft was now heading towards the mountainous countryside of the island of Honshu flying in a northerly direction. Mount Fuji, the highest mountain in Japan at 12,388 feet (3776 metres) lay only 15 miles away on their right. They then made a gentle turn to the northeasterly heading towards Yokota airfield used by the US Air Force, which lies to the northwest of the greater metropolis of Tokyo. The controller tried desperately to contact the aircraft as did the approach controller at Yokota thinking the aircraft may now be headed for that airfield but there was no reply.

The aircraft continued to make several turns, apparently at random, and was seen to make a very tight 360° turn whilst continuing to descend. Finally, on radar, the controller saw the aircraft straighten out on an easterly heading and when the radar paint showed the aircraft at a dangerously low 13,500 feet they heard the spine chilling call from the aircraft,

"JL123, JL123 – uncontrollable!"

The controller tried to assist the aircraft with a suggested switch of radio frequencies to Haneda Approach in preparation for a landing but the frantic reply of the crewmember was a request to "Stay with us". The descent continued to a very dangerous height of 9000 feet when the aircraft called again requesting a radar vector to Haneda.

The action on the flightdeck had been frenetic. The realisation that all flying controls were not functioning would cause the doughtiest of aircrew extreme concern but there was still a chance. As all pilots learn in their initial flying training by using asymmetric engine thrust they could make the aircraft turn, albeit slowly and uncomfortably and by using more or less power they had a small amount of control in pitch. They might be able to control their descent to a safe, but probably very rough, landing. Electric flap operation could also be used to further assist the pitch control. They still did not know the cause of the decompression or the reason for the catastrophic loss of hydraulic fluid but all was soon to become clear.

A call from the cabin told them that all the oxygen masks had dropped. Almost immediately another call came to tell the flightcrew that damage had occurred towards the rear of the aircraft. The flight engineer understood that the baggage hold may have collapsed and that there was a problem with door right 5, the aft door on the right of the aircraft. This information was not strictly correct but it gave some clues as to the severity of the problem.

He asked the cabin crewmember making the call whether everyone was using their oxygen masks and rang off. He passed this information to the Captain advising that an emergency descent would be advisable. He was right but with little or no control and the aircraft lurching around alarmingly, that was easier said than done. The aircraft nose fell, they descended rapidly and the airspeed quickly increased which probably caused the subsequent pitch up and rapid climb with the airspeed now falling dangerously low. The instability was getting worse and there was little they could do. They certainly had little time to answer the radio calls from the anxious controller on the ground.

Slowly but surely the pilots regained a semblance of control over the huge height excursions and it was then that the Flight Engineer realised that they had failed, in the chaotic situation, to don their oxygen masks. This undoubtedly had caused mild hypoxia at the altitude they were at and the mind dulling effect of lack of oxygen had not helped them deal with the multiple emergencies on hand. He reminded the Captain and all crewmembers promptly donned their oxygen masks. They immediately found that they were better able to control the alarming gyrations of the crippled aircraft.

Their control problems were still far from ideal and with the copilot still hand flying, the Captain directed his efforts to control the speed and height. The Flight Engineer suggested that lowering the undercarriage, needed eventually for landing anyway, might stabilise the aircraft but the speed was such that it could be damaged if

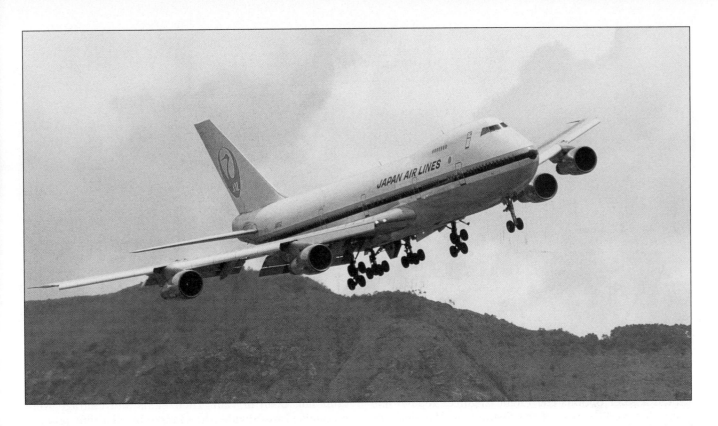

A JAL 747-200 on finals for the old Kai Tak airport at Hong Kong. In this accident the airliner had lost its entire vertical fin and some of the horizontal tailplane, rendering it essentially uncontrollable. (Rob Finlayson)

lowered immediately. As the gyrations reduced though the Flight Engineer took the opportunity when the speed was momentarily quite low, to select the undercarriage down. The resultant change of trim required immediate correction with thrust but the move was successful.

The increased drag stopped the fairly violent pitch changes, which were causing huge and uncontrolled speed and height variations but it also reduced their ability to steer the aircraft with asymmetric thrust. The aircraft now commenced a 360° turn to the right. Gradually they regained control and were now in a fairly steady descent and miraculously headed towards Haneda Airport, albeit with the aircraft continuously rolling from side to side. The cabin crew, on their own initiative, were briefing the passengers for an emergency landing. Whatever had happened the cabin and passengers had been prepared for the worst.

The few moments of relatively good control of the aircraft were short lived and despite using the landing gear and discussing the use of flaps, the aircraft now had a mind of its own with little the crew could do to control height or direction. They were now below 9000 feet and heading towards the mountainous countryside in central Honshu.

The Captain sighted a mountain dead ahead and called for a turn to the right. The application of power was nullified by the drag of the undercarriage and they continued down. The Captain called again, more urgently, for a turn to the right. Adding more power the aircraft again became very unstable and the nose pitched violently up. The aircraft climbed 2000 feet virtually out of control while the airspeed fell to 120 knots, right on the stalling speed.

"Maximum power" shouted the Captain with great urgency. The copilot acknowledged, 'firewalling' the thrust levers.

"Keep trying!" the Captain shouted. It wasn't clear what more the copilot could do.

The violent and necessary application of power had now totally destabilised the aircraft and the oscillations resumed. The crew continued their desperate efforts to regain control and maintain a safe altitude and airspeed, the Captain issuing urgent instructions, which were valiantly carried out by the First Officer. No command training should be this bad!

The violent climbs and wild speed excursions continued for several minutes activating the stall warning and evoking even more desperate calls from the Captain. The violent movements of the aircraft with its very sluggish and unpredictable response to the power changes finally took its toll; it was impossible to time the power changes to effect the desired movement of the aircraft. They did manage to get the aircraft climbing once more but it gradually turned to the northwest once again towards the mountains of central Honshu. It was 6.51pm, they had been fighting the stricken aircraft for 26 minutes with various degrees of success, but it was still flying. The radio calls from Tokyo and Yokota had to be ignored, there was no time to think let alone reply.

The controller noted that the aircraft was again climbing and hoped that the crew had regained some control of their altitude in this area of high ground. He was not aware of the continuing and dramatic events in the cockpit. "Nose up, nose up" would be immediately followed with "Nose down, nose down" from the Captain. He tried to extend flaps but they would not operate, however, he succeeded on the alternate operating system. At 6.53 the Captain called Tokyo as they climbed back to 12,000 feet,

"JL123 uncontrol, JL123 uncontrol" the message was clear as was the hidden cry for help.

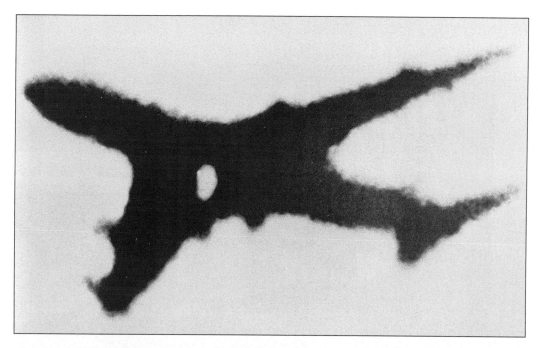

A chance photograph snapped by an amateur at long range but clear enough to show the extent of damage suffered by JL123 that day. Photos like this are a great asset to the investigative air crash specialists. (Arrow Books/Associated Press)

Tokyo control passed their distance to Haneda and advised them that Yokota was also available if that presented a safer option. The Flight Engineer replied and asked for confirmation of the distance to Haneda. The time was 6.55 pm.

The control difficulties were becoming worse by the minute and the crew frantically fought to retain, rather than regain, control. The following transcript from the cockpit voice recorder with aircraft performance data from the flight recorder speaks for itself.

6.54.40 – CAPTAIN: Nose up! (Aircraft climbs once more to a peak of just over 10,000 feet – airspeed falls off to 160 knots)

6.54.47 – CAPTAIN: Nose down! Down to the limit!

6.54.55 – CAPTAIN: Flap all!

6.55.04 – COPILOT: Yes – flap ten.

6.55.15 – CAPTAIN: Nose up! (aircraft enters steep descending turn to the right, airspeed increases to 200 knots

6.55.17 – CAPTAIN: Nose up!

6.55.19 – CAPTAIN: Nose up! (Steep turn continues – aircraft descending fast at 2000 feet per minute)

6.55.25 – CAPTAIN: Nose up!

6.55.42 – CAPTAIN: Hey – halt the flap! (Airspeed is falling sharply again)

6.55.48 – CAPTAIN: Ah... don't lower the flap so much.

6.55.50 – CAPTAIN: Flap up... Flap up... Flap up!

6.55.52 – ENGINEER: Flap up!

6.55.53 – CAPTAIN: Flap up!

6.55.54 – COPILOT: Yes.

6.55.55 – CAPTAIN: Power! Power!

6.55.57 – CAPTAIN: Flap!

6.55.58 – COPILOT It's up!

6.55.59 – CAPTAIN: Nose up! Nose up... Power! (Aircraft has turned about 200° to the right – descending turn continues to tighten)

6.56.14 – GPWS: (Ground Proximity Warning System) Sink rate...

6.56.15 – GPWS: Sink rate... pull up... pull up... pull up... pull up...

(Continues to sound the same warning)

6.56.25 – (Sound of aircraft striking trees) GPWS: Pull up... pull up... pull up...

6.56.28 – (Sound of aircraft impacting mountainside).

Sadly the valiant efforts of the crew to save the aircraft had been in vain. Their skills and courage were recognised worldwide and admired by all airline pilots.

American investigators, having determined the cause of the accident, could not believe that the crew had kept the aircraft flying for so long. Captain Mitsuo Nakano, JAL'S deputy chief Boeing 747 pilot, commented that "In spite of being in such a terrible plight, the aircraft was kept in the air on engine thrust only. That is an incredible performance". Captain Homer Mouden of the US Flight Safety Foundation agreed. "The crew exhibited great courage and skill in trying to keep it flying" he stated. It seems unjust that on this occasion, the crewmembers were not rewarded for their efforts. But that is not the end of the story.

The aircraft had finally crashed near the top of the 5400 foot high Mount Osutaka flying headlong into the pine covered slopes. The first to the scene was a helicopter, which reported the total devastation, many spot fires and that there was, understandably, no sign of any survivors. The crash site was extremely remote, steep and very narrow mountain tracks provided the only access to the terrible scene.

Rescuers and crash investigators would have a very difficult job reaching the site. It was 14 hours after the crash that the first firemen and civil defence workers reached the site. To add to their trouble the weather had deteriorated, the aircraft had been broken apart on impact and pieces were scattered over a large area. There was practically no hope of finding any survivors.

Miracles do happen though and, as a fireman stood on the steep slopes surveying the unpleasant job ahead of them, he saw movement, an arm waving. A young woman was quickly released from the wreckage surrounding her and was able to give her name before she was winched gently into a rescue helicopter; Yumi Ochiai had her personal miracle that day. Then, to their amazement, the rescuers found a schoolgirl wedged in a tree with only minor injuries. This discovery was quickly followed by them finding a young woman and her daughter covered with pieces of aircraft wreckage.

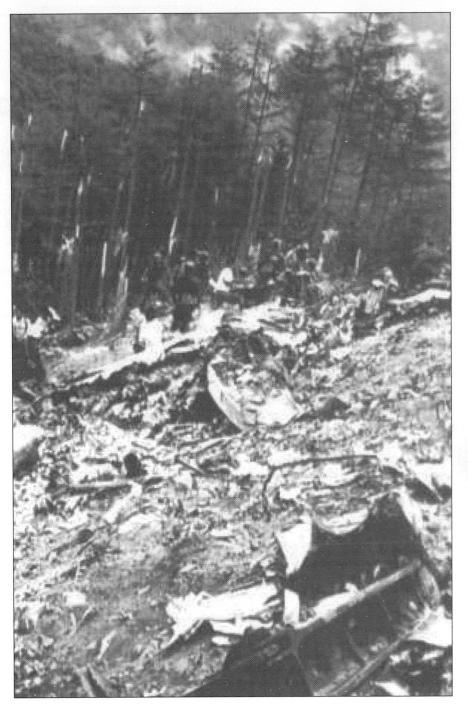

All of these survivors had been seated towards the rear of the aircraft, a curious factor in many accidents. Sadly no other passengers were found alive but Yumi was able to provide a valuable account of exactly what had taken place at the time of the decompression, which gave the investigators some important clues.

By another amazing coincidence, an amateur photographer had taken a shot of the stricken aircraft minutes before it crashed. From this photograph it became clear that severe damage had occurred in the tail section and that the fin, which gives directional stability to the aircraft, was almost totally missing. Not only had the pilots to deal with the loss of control with the hydraulic failure, but there was little doubt that the continuous rolling and lurching had been aggravated by the missing fin. It made their efforts even more remarkable. This photograph was another important clue to the cause of the disaster and set the investigators off on the trail of the missing fin; Lady Luck was on their side!

A Japanese Maritime Self-Defence Force destroyer coincidentally came across some floating wreckage on Sagami Bay, many miles from the crash site. It included a large piece of the fin floating on the surface. Close examination of the parts revealed that they had sustained damage before being detached from the aircraft and this concentrated the investigation of the initial cause of the disaster to this area of the aircraft. The location of the find gave strong evidence that the fin of the aircraft had probably separated at the time of the decompression.

Having found the suspect 'right 5' door, in the wreckage still firmly locked in place; the failure of that door was eliminated from the enquiry. The enquiry began to focus on the rear pressure bulkhead, which had been severely damaged but was being meticulously pieced together.

The cause was finally determined to be the failure of a repair to part of the rear pressure bulkhead, which had permitted a sudden rush of pressurised air to enter the unpressurised cavities inside the tailplane. This had literally blown off most of the fin and taken out hydraulic lines causing the total hydraulic failure. It had resulted from a small developing crack, which, due to its inaccessibility, had gone unnoticed in the regular and thorough checks, which were routinely performed by JAL.

It is not the purpose of this story to recount the full findings of the investigators, that is a matter of record. The purpose is to give credit to all the crew of this flight who performed valiantly and with incredible skill in the most stressful situation that can be imagined and further to record the safety advances that resulted from the painstaking investigation.

The basic design and structure of the magnificent Boeing aircraft were found to be without fault as were their preproduction testing procedures. Nonetheless Boeing made several major changes to the design in order to counter any repetition of this once in a million failure. The safety of the travelling public had been further improved but at a terrible cost.

The conversations on the flightdeck and the aircraft's flight characteristics were derived from the cockpit voice recorder transcript and from the transcript of the flight data recorder commonly known as the black box.

CHAPTER TEN

Captain, My Captain

Everyone who has ever flown will know about seat belts and when they are to be fastened and when not. The public address announcements when seat belts are required vary though. Sometimes you may hear "... fasten your seatbelt loosely..." in the announcement.

You could not have had worse advice since, in the event of severe turbulence a loosely fastened seatbelt may cause worse injuries than no seat belt at all. This is a story about a loosely fastened seatbelt and the dire and dramatic consequences that resulted.

It was a hazy June morning, cool but promising to be a fine day over central England when British Airways flight BA 5390 prepared to depart from Birmingham Airport for Malaga in Spain. These 'bucket & spade' flights, as they were known in the trade, were usually full of holidaymakers heading for one of the many sunny and popular resorts on the continent. For the crews they were very routine flights, usually to airports they knew well and home for dinner. In the cabin it sometimes got a bit lively but the excellent BA flight attendants were well able to deal with any over exuberant passengers and to give assurance to any first time flyers who may be nervous.

Captain Tim Lancaster was in command of the BAC 111 twinjet and supported by his First Officer Alastair Atchison. At 42 years old, Captain Lancaster had accumulated over 11,000 hours of experience mostly in long haul operations. His F/O was also highly experienced with over 1000 hours on this aircraft type alone. Purser John Heward was in charge of the cabin supervising the three other cabin crew, all that was needed on this relatively small short haul aircraft which that day had 81 passengers.

The flight made a normal departure from Birmingham with the F/O at the controls and set off in a southerly direction across southwest England climbing gradually out of the haze into clear skies. The airline traffic in Europe is very dense and Britain is no exception. They were under close radar control from the moment they departed with various clearances to climb higher as they cleared crossing traffic. As they transferred to the Bristol Sector Controller of London Air Traffic Control they were further steered around other traffic and cleared to climb to Flight Level 230 (23,000 feet).

Having flown the aircraft by hand in the early stages of the flight, the F/O had then engaged the autopilot which, according to company procedures, was now being operated by the Captain. With the autopilot engaged and operating normally the pilots were able to relax and release their shoulder harnesses, always worn for take-off and landing. The Captain also loosened the lap strap of his harness for comfort's sake.

In the cabin, with the seatbelt sign now off, the cabin crew were preparing for the meal service. They had only departed 13 minutes earlier but it was essential on these flights to get the service underway early, there could always be periods of 'tea time turbulence' when they would have to suspend meal service.

The aircraft was climbing through 17,300 feet on its way to an interim cruise level of 23,000 feet when there was a noise like a massive explosion in the cockpit. It was total chaos as dust and equipment momentarily flew around the cockpit together with bits of debris.

The cause of the noise was not apparent back in the cabin but its effects were immediately obvious. Ears popped and the cabin filled with a white mist, the classic phenomena associated with an explosive decompression. Looking forward the passengers and stewards could see that the cockpit door had been blown in and its shattered remains were lying inside the cockpit across the centre control pedestal covering the communication equipment and the throttles, seriously hindering the operation of the aircraft.

Steward Nigel Ogden had been in the cabin by the cockpit door when the decompression occurred and he was thrown violently into the cockpit with the remains of the door by the blast of air.

Even more alarmingly he could see that the Captain had been drawn out through the gaping hole and was only prevented from being sucked out of the aircraft altogether by his legs which were trapped between his seat, the flight controls and the window frame.

As he recovered himself from the shock of his sudden fall he looked up and had a close up view of the cause of the problem; the Captain's number one cockpit window (the window immediately in front of him) had blown out and was totally missing! Even more alarmingly he could see that the Captain had been drawn out through the gaping hole and was only prevented from being sucked out of the aircraft altogether by his legs which were trapped between his seat, the flight controls and the window frame. The slipstream was also pinning his upper body to the top of the fuselage outside the aircraft! Only the Captain's lower torso was still inside the cockpit.

Ogden leapt forward and grasped the Captain with a 'rugby grip' around the waist and legs and hung on for dear life. Despite his best efforts though he could not pull the Captain back in and had a strong impression that he was slowly being sucked further out.

Captain Lancaster was still conscious but had no idea of what had occurred. All he knew was that he couldn't breathe, the slipstream was so overpowering. He found that by turning his head slightly to one side he was able to take a few breaths. As he did so he found he was looking directly at the T shaped tail of the aircraft and

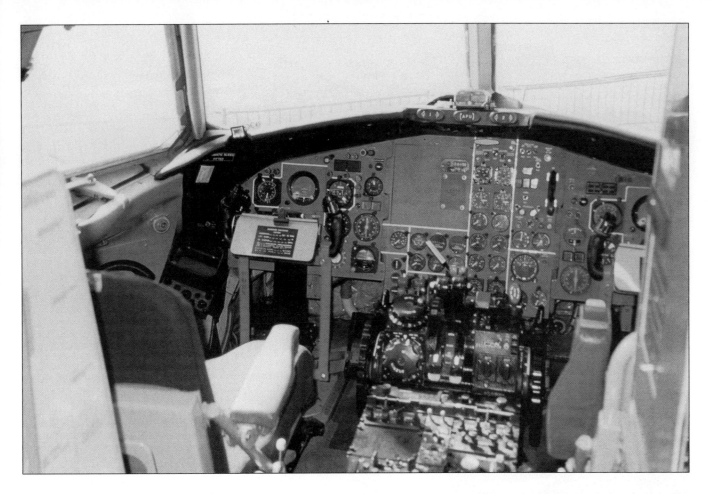

The cockpit of a BAC-111 showing the captain's seat and the centre pedestal. Forward and to the left of the captain's seat is the window which failed and through which the captain was sucked. (Jim Thorn)

could see the razor thin radio aerial which ran from the top of the fuselage to the tail. He felt that he was 'glued' to the top of the aircraft by the slipstream – more than 300mph with the aircraft still at cruise speed!

The First Officer who had been adjusting his heading bug to the latest radar steer, was hit hard on the left shoulder by a section of the shattered cockpit door. Already partially disorientated by the sudden explosive noise of the window blowing out and the effects of the subsequent decompression, he was now faced with a triple emergency; the decompression, incapacitation of his fellow pilot and the aircraft was starting to enter a spiral dive under full climb power.

The autopilot had been disconnected as the Captain struck the control column during his traumatic partial exit from the aircraft and nothing was controlling the aircraft, on top of everything else they were on the brink of a jet upset. Unbeknownst to him the autopilot master switch had also been knocked out preventing its re-engagement should he want to use it. The First Officer immediately took over control and hand flew the aircraft back to level flight but could not reach the throttles with the wrecked cockpit door all over the central control panel. He finally managed to squeeze his left hand under the debris and reduce the engine power preparatory to an emergency descent.

The noise of rushing air from the gaping hole where the window had been made things doubly difficult. Atchison broadcast a distress call but could not be sure if it had been heard; he certainly could not hear any

reply. He had to get the aircraft to a lower altitude since they were well above the safe height to be without oxygen but not so high that it was immediately imperative.

The Purser, John Heward, rushed into the cockpit responding to the frantic shouts of the First Officer quickly clearing the remains of the shattered cockpit door from the throttles then taking a firm grip on Nigel Ogden to prevent both him and the Captain being sucked out of the window. In the cabin the remaining crew instructed passengers to fasten their seatbelts and, taking their emergency stations, tried to reassure them that all would be well.

First Officer Atchison was finally able to put the aircraft into an emergency descent and elected not to waste time or to distract his efforts by simultaneously putting on his mask. Without the mask on he would also be able to shout instructions to the cabin crew. It was fortunate that the aircraft was still at a relatively low altitude when the emergency occurred, he could quickly return the aircraft to a safer level. None the less, he had to complete all the normal procedures from memory without the benefit of the normal challenge and reply checklist calls between the two pilots.

On the ground the controller did not know what had happened. He knew the aircraft was descending, that was plain on his radar screen. It was to be some time before two way communications could be re-established and the magnitude of the problems would become clear to him.

First Officer Atchison, having descended to a safe altitude, was well aware that the speed of the aircraft

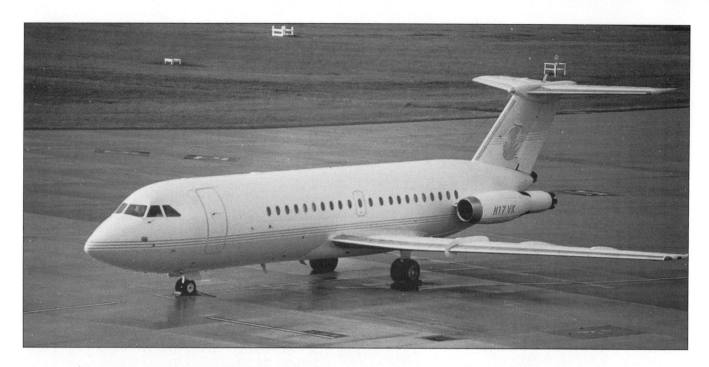

A BAC-111 similar to the one in this incident. The window which failed is the front cockpit window on the left side in this photo. (George Pergaminelis)

(below) Captain Tim Lancaster and purser John Heward.

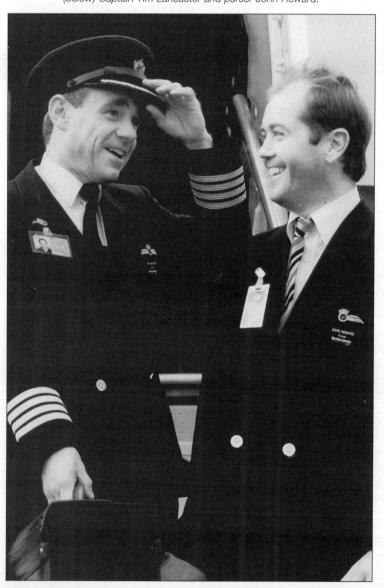

was causing great difficulties for the Captain's rescuers, let alone the Captain. Having dispensed with two emergencies, was now able to slow the aircraft and reduce the drag on the Captains body. He had obviously already sustained multiple injuries but slowing the aircraft would reduce the terrible flailing of his limbs and upper torso.

The necessary and well intentioned slowing of the aircraft reduced the slipstream's effect on the Captain and his upper torso now slid down from the top of the fuselage. Only Ogden and Heward now held the Captain's whole body weight. Cabin Steward Simon Rogers, having cleared away the remaining debris from the cockpit door, came back into the flight deck and secured himself with the seatbelt of the empty cockpit observer's seat behind the Captain.

He could see that the Captain's back was now bent back the wrong way around the windscreen pillar, it presented a grotesque and worrying sight to him and would make recovery even more difficult. Nonetheless he lent two more hands to the task of stopping the Captain sliding further from the aircraft and trying to get him back inside. They could all see the Captain through the other cockpit window but still the force of the slipstream made the task of recovery impossible. It looked as if he was simply lying on the side of the aircraft, still pinioned there by the slipstream.

Nigel Ogden, who had now been pulled very close to the frame of the missing window, was suffering too as he was buffeted against the icy cold frame of the window and was starting to get frostbite. The injuries and effort were fast sapping his strength and it was taking all the efforts of two people just to hold on, if they failed or relaxed their efforts, even for a moment, there was little doubt the Captain would die. With Simon Rogers now holding onto Captain Lancaster, Nigel

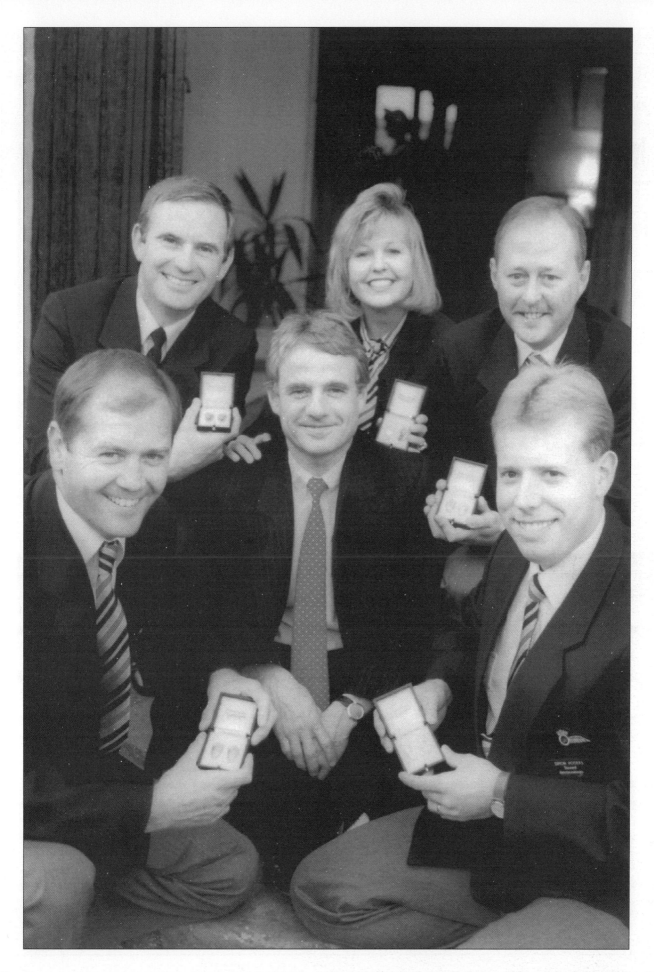

All smiles and well deserved – top left clockwise – Alastair Aitcheson, Sue Prince, Nigel Ogden, Simon Rogers, Tim Lancaster and John Heward.

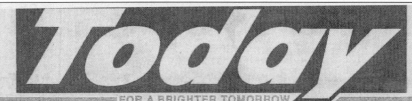

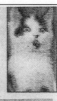

BOMBED

DRAMATIC PICTURES
PAGES 4 & 5

INSURE YOUR PET FREE

See page 11

FOR A BRIGHTER TOMORROW

Jet saved as crew grab pilot sucked out of window

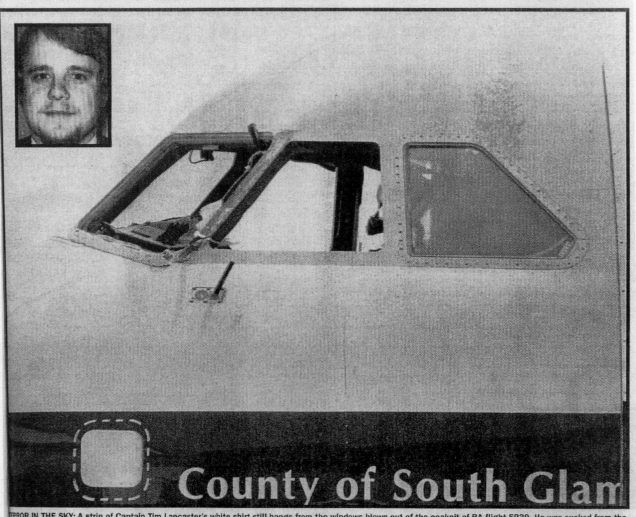

County of South Glam

TERROR IN THE SKY: A strip of Captain Tim Lancaster's white shirt still hangs from the windows blown out of the cockpit of BA flight 5930. He was sucked from the centre window and battered against the one on right, stained with his blood. Captain Lancaster (inset) was not dragged inside until the aircraft landed 13 minutes later

HEROES AT 23,000 FEET

A PILOT sucked through an airliner's cockpit window at 23,000 ft was saved by the courage of his crew.

Captain Tim Lancaster was pulled halfway out of the window of BA flight 5390 when two screens blew out on a trip from Birmingham to Spain.

Steward Nigel Ogden, 36, dived onto the flight deck and as the captain was disappearing into space, grabbed his legs.

Colleague Simon Rogers, 29, rushed to help and strapped himself into the captain's seat to give him extra support. Co-pilot Alistair Atchinson put the plane in to a dive and made a perfect emergency landing within 13 minutes.

The 41-year-old captain's blood-stained clothes were ripped off by the roaring winds. He suffered fractured

Turn to Page 20

Dramatic photo showing the missing window and remains of blood on the fuselage where Captain Lancaster was constantly pummelled against the airframe by the savage slipstream for some 13 minutes. (Today)

Ogden was able to release his tiring hold on the Captain and return to the cabin to be treated by Stewardess Sue Prince.

Despite the best efforts of the three stewards combined they had been unable to draw the Captain back inside the cockpit but they did manage to prevent him slowly, inch by inch, being drawn further out of the aircraft. The relieving steward was now holding only the Captain's ankles he had slid so far out of the window, it was a desperate fight against time. The effort of holding onto the Captain was now telling on them.

The lower speed also reduced the terrible wind noise in the flightdeck and two way communications were now re-established with the ground. The F/O was finally able, to the utter amazement of the ground controller, to confirm the Mayday situation, pass the full and dramatic nature of their emergency and to request radar vectors to the nearest aerodrome which turned out to be Southampton.

He had no time to navigate or tune beacons; documents carried in the cockpit showing approach data to Southampton's runways would simply blow away, radar guidance all the way in was essential. The controller, Chris Rundle, provided him with all the data that he needed to be assured that he could land the aircraft safely on the relatively short runway at this small regional airport and gave him continual radar vectors to make an approach to the duty runway. His very professional aid greatly assisted Atchison in his dilemma.

The thoughts in the Captain's mind can only be imagined. Not knowing what was preventing him sliding totally out of the aircraft, he was facing a death plunge from a great height. Finally the trauma caused him to pass in and out of consciousness. In the brief periods of consciousness he could see fields and cars below him but thankfully, before long, he passed out completely and was unable to further contemplate his fate or feel further pain or buffeting.

Completing all the prelanding cockpit checks and drills from memory the First Officer flew the aircraft down the approach path. Knowing that a firm or heavy landing might finally cause the weight of the Captain's body to jerk itself free from the rescuers' hands, the First Officer concentrated all his efforts on a smooth touchdown but a gentle deceleration on this short runway was out of the question. The BAC 111 landed smoothly and he brought the aircraft to a stop within 900 metres being as easy on the brakes as he dared within the constraints of the runway.

The Captain was now hanging vertically from the window but the strength of the cabin crew was drained and they still could not drag him back inside the aircraft. It was not until the airport fire and rescue staff drew their truck alongside the cockpit window and combined with other members of the rescue team, who had now entered the cockpit and were not fatigued by the long struggle, that they were able to lift him gently back through the window frame.

He was carried out and put on a stretcher, now partially conscious again, and transported to Southampton General Hospital. As he slowly regained full consciousness he could not understand why he was in hospital or fully remember what had happened. He remembered going to work and wondered if he had had a car accident on the way!

From the moment of the decompression until the safe landing it had been 22 minutes of stark terror for the Captain, frantic effort for the stewards and 22 minutes of mighty endeavour for the First Officer. He had had to coordinate the cabin crew, fly the aeroplane and land safely, all the time having to carefully judge his actions to ensure the safety of the aircraft and passengers and, at the same time, trying to prevent further injury to the Captain – a delicate balancing act.

There had been no simulator training for this emergency, it required quick thinking and superlative airmanship greatly assisted by the cabin crew who acted with alacrity, resourcefulness and courage. The Captain was indeed fortunate to have such a good team on his aircraft that day.

Amazingly, despite the terrible battering he had taken in the slipstream, Captain Lancaster only had bone fractures in his right arm and wrist, a broken left thumb, much bruising, frostbite and, not surprisingly, was suffering from shock. The worst injury was damage to nerve tissue in his upper arms which cost him the use of his arms for over three months. He finally made a full recovery.

The stewards who had valiantly hung on to him throughout the incident had a few cuts and bruises but were otherwise uninjured. The passengers suffered no ill effects apart from an understandable fright and a slight delay to the start of their holidays. It certainly gave them something to talk about when they finally arrived in Malaga!

The brilliant airmanship and conduct of the whole crew was duly recognised. The Queen's Commendation for Valuable Services in the Air was awarded to First Officer Atchison and to Purser John Heward, Stewards Nigel Ogden and Simon Rogers and to Stewardess Sue Prince. International recognition came from the Federation Aeronautique Internationale who awarded First Officer Atchison and the whole cabin crew the Diploma for Outstanding Airmanship. They also received the Hugh Gordon-Burge Memorial Award from the Guild of Air Pilots and Navigators. First Officer Atchison was presented with the Polaris Medal from the International Federation of Airline Pilots, the Gold Medal from the British Airline Pilots' Association and the Master's Medal from GAPAN.

British Airways presented the entire crew with the Award of Excellence. These awards from this array of august bodies truly represent the immense admiration of the aviation world for the airmanship and skill of the First Officer and the courage of the whole crew. Their best reward was undoubtedly the knowledge that they had saved a life and brought the aircraft safely home.

Note by author – this account was greatly assisted by the personal recollections of Captain Lancaster and First Officer Atchison.

CHAPTER ELEVEN

No Parachutes!

What happens to ageing airliners when they become too expensive to maintain and uneconomical for normal airline operations?

Many such aircraft are simply sold for scrap. In America they are parked in serried ranks in the Mojave Desert where they deteriorate more slowly in the bone dry desert air. It was from just such a 'park' that a group of Australian aviation enthusiasts recovered a Super Constellation and after years of work, trans Pacific commuting and hunting for hard to get spare parts, restored it to its original airworthy condition and the Qantas livery of its era. The desert air had not seriously affected the aircraft structure but the bird colonies which had taken up residence had caused considerable damage and the recovery team spent weeks meticulously removing layers of guano!

The more ancient machines are also unattractive to the flying public and that alone can reduce airline revenue as customers move to airlines flying newer models. Some older aircraft, which have been well maintained during their airline life, are snapped up by airfreight operators for a song and have made many a fortune for their new owners. This story is about one such Boeing 707, the first of the commercially successful big jets.

Originally purchased by Pan American when the Boeing 707 was 'state of the art' this aircraft served with Iran Air, Uganda Airways and Dan Air, a small airline in the UK before being converted to a freighter. It was then extensively used on the North Atlantic freight runs by a series of operators and, in between owners, spent much time in outdoor storage at a number of lightly used aerodromes in the south of England which undoubtedly did little for its preservation or condition. Now over 30 years old and with 60,000 hours of service to its credit, this ageing 707 was purchased by the Nigerian airfreight company Trans-Air Ltd for charter freight operations to the African continent and was based in Luxembourg. It was from Luxembourg that it departed on the fateful flight.

In March 1992, in a plain white and silver livery with the name Kabo Air Charter emblazoned on the cargo door, flight QNK 671 was to take a heavy load of 40 tons of mining equipment to Lagos for the Esso oil company flying on to Ghana and Mali and then, as further freight contracts arose, to other ports of call – virtually a roving commission after the first few stops.

As with many such operators, it was a cosmopolitan crew that manned the aircraft that day. Captain Ingemar Bergelund, a Swedish national, had logged 25,000 hours and flown the 707 for the last 10 years, experience that was to prove invaluable. The First Officer and the Flight Engineer were British. F/O Martin Emery had 16,500 hours flying time in his logbook, at least half of that on multi engined jet aircraft. E/O Terry Boone, with over 18,000 hours on 707 aircraft alone, was undoubtedly the most experienced of all the crewmembers on the type. They were very familiar with the long haul cargo operations and had, in recent weeks, done several such flights together around the African continent.

To carry out the cargo loading and unloading operations and to maintain and service the aircraft 'on the run', since there often being no reliable maintenance facilities or staff at many of the airfields they visited, the crew included Loadmaster Ingebar Einarrsen, a thoroughly professional operator who hailed from Iceland and the highly qualified Nigerian Ground Engineer Nwabadike. Both jobs were not easy, especially in the heat and dust of most African airfields with the quality of the ground staff ever suspect. Good humour and an ability to carry on in adverse circumstances were essential qualities which both these men possessed in abundance.

The takeoff from Luxembourg was, by all accounts, spectacular. Despite the relatively cool March day and the early model Pratt & Whitney JT3D-3b engines at full takeoff power, the acceleration of the heavily laden 707 down the 4000 metre Luxembourg runway was slow. For any full power takeoff in the early model 707s it was common place for the compressor speeds to be on their upper limits, the engine exhaust gas temperatures (EGT) on the 'red line' – today was no exception.

Most crews doubted that they would ever stop on the runway from a V_1 abort of the takeoff but Pratt & Whitney thankfully built very reliable engines. At 7.15am they lifted off for their African Odyssey using, as the saying goes, 'every inch of the runway'!

Raising the gear and taking advantage of a slight fall away in the ground at the end of the runway, they brought their flaps in as quickly as possible to accelerate to their best climb speed. The 707 when at top weight, always performed much better in the climb at the top end of the speed range. They were cleared to climb without restriction to their first planned cruise level of Flight Level 290 (29,000 feet) and given direct tracking to Saint

They were now in a life threatening multiple emergency situation. The height at which the 707 could maintain level flight on two engines was well below the mountainous countryside below them, with two engines failed they had lost half their electrical supply, half the pressure air to maintain cabin pressure and most of the aircraft hydraulic systems had failed.

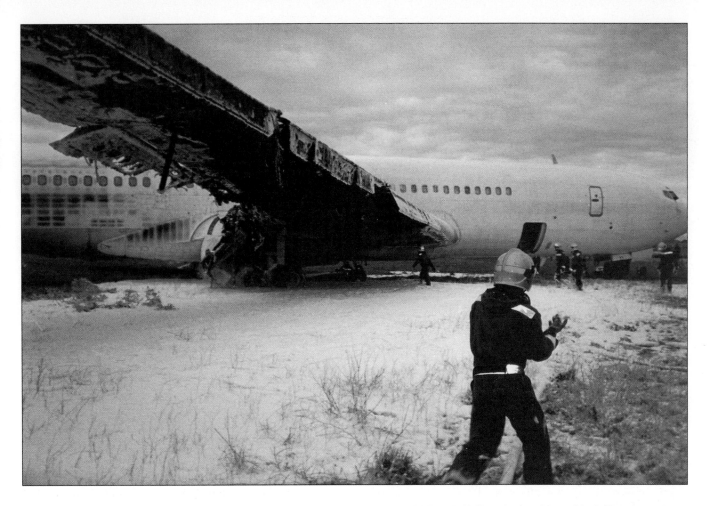

Missing both right side engines, the battered 707 lies in a sea of foam at the French Air Force base at Istres. (Martin Emery)

Prex VOR which cut out many small turns and again improved their sluggish rate of climb. It took them nearly one hour to reach their cruise level by which time they had crossed the Swiss border and, levelling off, they had established the aircraft at the cruise speed of Mach .80. The planned flightpath now headed them in a southerly direction towards Martigues and across the Alps.

The combination of high ground and the strong upper winds can often cause the phenomena of 'mountain waves', similar to a giant sea swell, which at best can make speed and altitude control difficult and, at worst, can cause severe turbulence. They had no indication of turbulent clouds on the weather radar but, as they approached the Alps, turbulence began and steadily increased in intensity until, as the F/O later commented it became "As rough as hell".

The crew hunkered down for the rough ride, putting on the full safety harness and reducing the cruise speed to the Boeing recommended speed for severe turbulence of Mach .78. The Captain very professionally, although the autopilot was engaged with 'altitude lock', kept his hands on the control column. In extreme turbulence the early model autopilots systems could drop out, even in 'turb' mode, and often did not handle significant turbulence well. It sometimes became necessary to hand fly the aircraft. Ahead of them, not far from their planned track, lay much high ground including the highest peak in Europe, Mont Blanc, reaching 15,771 feet above sea level, just under 14,000 feet below their cruise level.

It was inadvisable to climb higher if the turbulence

extended to higher levels but, having no reports of the ride at higher altitudes and in case they could clear the rough air, they asked for a climb to 33,000 feet. They were quite heavy for that climb but slowly and surely they inched their way higher under their clearance from air traffic control. The 707 continued to be thrown about and the crew observed all the classic signs of a rough ride in the aircraft.

The wings flexed up and down and the engine 'pods' danced from side to side. Alarming when viewed by passengers but all a design feature of the aircraft which actually gave it greater strength in the circumstances. Gradually the dark cloud thinned and they had glimpses of clear sky above so there was a good chance they would be 'in the clear' and have a smoother ride at their new altitude.

The amber light and warning tone indicating 800 feet to go to the new altitude had just sounded in the cockpit when there were two enormous thuds and the aircraft shook violently. The intensity of the noise and the unmistakable shudder that was felt by all the crew was immediately followed by a rapid roll into a 45° bank and a different, aerodynamic buffeting indicating that they were right on the stall, highly dangerous at this high altitude and at the aircraft's limiting weight.

The 45° bank alone was enough to increase their small margin over stall, immediate and correct action was required. It all happened so quickly that before the Captain could correct the flightpath the bank angle had reached a staggering 55°.

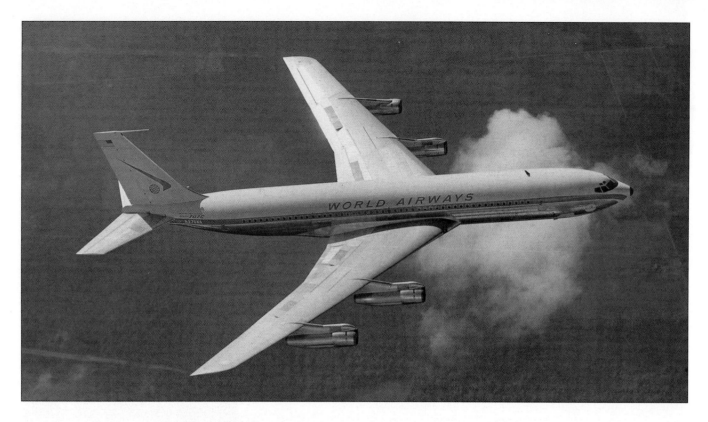

A Boeing 707-300 series jetliner identical to the one in this story. (Boeing)

The Captain disconnected the autopilot and applied full controls to regain level flight. Before his struggle to regain control could be effective the situation on the flightdeck further deteriorated with the strident and deafening alarm of the fire warning bell. Coupled with the autopilot disconnect warning warbler and ominous sounds of structural stress, it was a literal bedlam of noise. Attempts to silence the fire warning bell failed, the 'cancel' button simply had no effect. To make matters worse the cabin altitude warning horn started blaring telling the crew that the cabin pressure was failing which would require them to go on oxygen. There had been a catastrophic failure which had yet to be determined.

The Captain gradually fought the aircraft back to wings level but was unable to maintain altitude; the aircraft was now heading down fast. The two right hand thrust levers had jammed fully forward; he matched them with number one and two thrust levers attempting to get maximum power to arrest the descent. He suspected severe structural damage but was about to descend back into the turbulence, the safe speed for structural damage was considerably lower than that recommended speed for turbulence penetration, he had to make a decision.

He opted for keeping the aircraft in one piece and slowed down to 230 knots indicated airspeed which also allowed him to safely use full control deflection if he needed it. Fortunately the 707 was not 'fly by wire'. Even with loss of the hydraulic boost to the rudder it was possible to manoeuvre the aircraft although response was sluggish and the control pressure required to use the rudder was extremely heavy.

The axiom of good airmanship in an emergency is 'first fly the aircraft'. When control is regained then and only then start to deal with the emergencies. Number three and four fire warning lights had illuminated at the time of the first signs of trouble and now had to be actioned. The Captain called for the fire drill and engine shut down for number four engine and then number three ensuring that maximum power had been applied to the remaining two engines.

They were now in a life threatening multiple emergency situation. The height at which the 707 could maintain level flight on two engines was well below the mountainous countryside below them, with two engines failed they had lost half their electrical supply, half the pressure air to maintain cabin pressure and most of the aircraft hydraulic systems had failed. The double engine failure itself called for a landing as soon as possible.

As they completed the 'memory' emergency engine shutdown drills the F/O looked out of his side window to see if there was any visible sign of fire. He could not believe what he saw, or to be more correct, did not see. Despite being in cloud the wing was clearly visible and where the outboard, number four engine should have been there was nothing but a gaping hole in the leading edge of the wing. Not only had the engine detached itself but in doing so had taken the engine pylon with it wrenching out part of the wing structure itself. He turned to the Captain and reported the incredible news but suddenly had a second thought. There had been two thumps and both starboard engines had indicated a fire. He pressed his face close to the window and peered back – it was not easy to see the inboard engine from the cockpit window. He was just able to see similar damage to the wing where number three engine had been; it too had fallen from the aircraft causing severe damage to the wing.

"Both starboard engines have gone" he called out urgently.

The engineer, frantically working at his panel to get as many systems back on line as possible, was in no mood for frivolity but the F/O was quickly able to convince him that this was no joke.

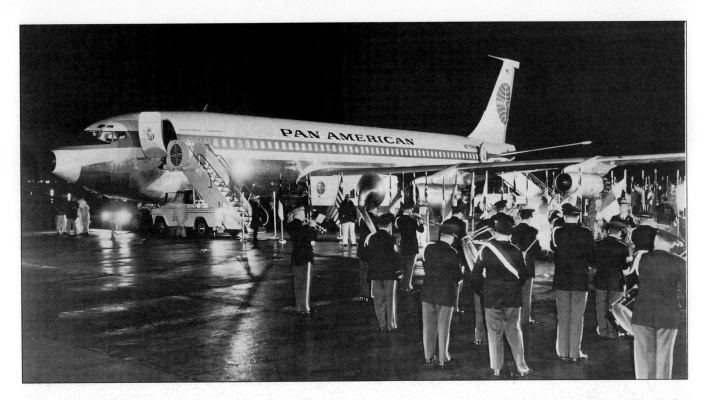

A moment in history as the inaugural Pan American World Airways 707 awaits passengers at Idlewild Airport, New York prior to making the first commercial trans Atlantic jet flight. Just as the emergence of the 707, and the competing Douglas DC-8 rendered the long range piston engined propliners obsolete, the emergence of the widebody 747 in the early seventies nowadays has the remnants of the 707 fleet configured as freighters and special mission aircraft. In the hands of third world operators though these ageing airliners are also sometimes maintained to less than first rate standards. (PanAm)

F/O Martin put out the Mayday call on the operating radio frequency requesting the Minimum Safe Altitude and radar vectors to the nearest aerodrome. Things went from bad to worse. Even though this call had been prefaced with the international Mayday distress call the controller, in broken English, simply asked for their position which, after their control problems and the erratic flight path of the aircraft, the F/O was hoping the controller could tell him. He enlarged that they had serious structural problems and very limited manoeuvrability but the controller seemed unable to grasp that the crew of this aircraft desperately needed help to relieve their workload which only he, the controller could give.

Added to this the continental controllers were never very fluent in the international language of aviation, English. Martin, hoping to impress upon the controller that there was an extreme emergency in progress, kept on transmitting the Mayday calls but was frustrated to get a series of directives to change frequency and to reselect the transponder code – extra and unnecessary work which they could well do without. The whole radio conversation was continually interrupted by other French speaking aircraft who, possibly being domestic flights, were not required to use or speak English and were not aware of the emergency in progress.

They should have been, Mayday is an international cry for help. The controller should have transferred all other aircraft off frequency so that he could devote his full attention to the problem in hand – he did not. Hoping to finally get the controller's full attention Martin backed up the Mayday calls by selecting the transponder to the Mayday code which would 'paint' a large, highly visible '7700' on the controllers screen which would also be seen by the supervising controller.

Up to this moment the crew had not cut off the fuel to the inboard failed engine hoping that they might be able to restart it and stop their inexorable descent towards the high ground (the Fire Switch, which had been pulled, does this automatically, but the checklist calls for the fuel shut off lever to be closed as well, as extra insurance). This was no longer an option and selecting the fuel shut off lever to 'closed', they cut the fuel supply to number three engine, or at least to where it had been. To their annoyance, the clamour of the fire warning bell continued to sound in the cockpit considerably hampering their vital flight deck communications.

With great presence of mind and realising that it was highly likely that they were not going to survive, Martin took out his camera and took a photograph of the starboard wing which would clearly show the missing engine and the damage it had caused in coming adrift. If they found the film in the wreckage at least the board of enquiry would have one clue as to what had happened.

Captain Bergelund continued to struggle with the aircraft controls but with 50% of the aircraft power not available, the descent could not be controlled. He just had to ensure that they kept a safe airspeed and try to navigate away from the high ground. That was easier said that done, they had had little time to tune radio beacons and there was still minimum help from control. Their intense workload and the gyrations of the aircraft had left them unsure of their exact position.

As they descended through 20,000 feet they broke out of the cloud and one of their problems was solved. Below them the vast and beautiful panorama of the Alps came into view. They would now be able to navigate visually around the higher peaks towards safer terrain but they still had to find an airport to bring the crippled

707 in for a safe landing. The Captain handed over control to the First Officer while he considered his options. They had a limited amount of time before they would run out of altitude!

At last help from the ground. They were given a southerly radar vector to Marseille-Marignane airport and passed the weather conditions there. The Captain ordered a fuel dump to reduce the aircraft weight for landing which would also improve their undesirably high rate of descent and give them more time. With the loss of half the hydraulic system they now had to lower the undercarriage using the manual hand cranks situated under hatches in the floor of the cockpit. This was a lengthy and arduous procedure.

As they neared Marseille airport it transpired that the approach to the duty runway was obscured by thunderstorms. Apart from the visibility problems they could not risk any further turbulence which would undoubtedly be present in and around the storms. The only alternative was to land downwind, which, with what was already going to be a high landing speed, was not a pleasant option. Martin set to work to see if there was not an alternative airport close enough for them to use. He knew there were several military aerodromes in the vicinity from his holiday flying in the area and scanned the air charts for the best option.

While he was doing this the Captain took back control of the aircraft as the other crew located the approach charts for Marseille and tuned up the radio beacons required for the approach. They were now down to 8000 and still descending, the remaining power not permitting them to maintain altitude. Normally the undercarriage, with the extra drag it caused, would have been lowered much later on an approach with only two engines but the lengthy manual lowering procedure required with the loss of one hydraulic system had forced their hand. The early extension was not helping their descent rate and, as with all two engine approaches, once it was down there was no chance of a successful go around if the approach was not spot on.

With hydraulic boost lost to the rudder and only the sheer brute force of one or both pilots' leg muscles to put in the required rudder deflection to keep the aircraft straight, they had to maintain a higher than desirable speed to keep the aircraft heading in the right direction, absolutely essential for the approach and landing. As they continued their difficult approach the F/O saw a huge airstrip through a break in the cloud. It was closer than Marseille and clear of any bad weather. He called the Marseille controller to find out which airfield it was. Luck was finally on their side. It was the military base of Istres, a flight test centre with a 4000 metre long runway and also used as an emergency landing place for the US space shuttles. They were handed over to Istres control.

To make their approach to Istres they had to turn to the left but against the rated power on the two left engines and despite superhuman efforts from the Captain, the aircraft would not turn to the left but was even starting to turn the other way. They had to make a sacrifice and the F/O reduced the power on the outboard left engine. This enabled them to start a very slow turn to the left towards the new haven. The thrust reduction once again increased their rate of descent and forced their hand. They would have to land downwind.

They now started to extend the flaps using the electrical flap extension system which immediately precipitated yet another dire emergency. Fuel had been escaping from the damaged fuel lines and tanks in the right wing. Combined with bare electrical wires left in the damaged area where number three engine had torn away the fuel ignited and caused a violent explosion. Most of the flaps were simply blown away damaging the elevator as the debris flew away in the slipstream causing further damage to the already fragile wing structure. The lack of flaps on the right hand side meant they now had asymmetric lift which made their directional control problem even more severe.

Smoke and flames poured from the right wing making a spectacular sight for the controllers in the Istres tower who now had the aircraft in sight. They twice radioed to tell the crew that the aircraft was on fire, of which the crew was only too well aware. Had they come this far only to perish in a fiery crash on the runway? The Captain held a slight bank to help maintain directional control and, heedless of the speed, they dived for the runway. The F/O adjusted the thrust to maintain their minimum control speed while the Captain, with a superhuman effort, physically aimed the aircraft at the landing point like a dart. An immediate landing was the only thing that was going to save them now. The tailwind was 30 knots, even with 4000 metres of runway they were going to be lucky to stop before the runway end.

Finally the wheels touched not far from the desired landing point. Normal braking had been lost with the hydraulics and the Captain reached for the pneumatic emergency brake handle. This system applied full braking with no modulation, there was no doubt they were going to blow most of their tyres causing more fires in the wheel wells. Applying short bursts of braking to try and preserve the tyres and using reverse thrust on the inboard engine only, they started to slow.

Miraculously the tyres held for a while allowing them to maintain control of the aircraft on the runway but they gradually lost directional control as what little rudder deflection they could achieve was lost and the tyres began to blow out. The aircraft slid off the runway onto the grass. Out of the corner of his eye the F/O saw vast clouds of thick black smoke and flames, the whole wing was now just a blazing inferno. They were going to have to make a very quick exit once they stopped.

The aircraft slithered across the grass finishing up at 90° to the runway heading and came to rest just short of a large sign which carried the message "DO NOT PASS THIS POINT"! The irony did not strike them at the time!

Realising that he was the only one who had seen the severity of the inferno out on the wing, as they came to a stop Martin shouted urgently for the Engineer to cut all fuel and electrics and opening his side window, he released the escape rope stowed above the window. This rope was fitted to allow crews to escape directly from the cockpit without entering the cabin.

"Evacuate, evacuate" he screamed. The other crewmembers needed little encouragement; out the windows and down the ropes they went. In the cabin the other two crewmembers made their own exit and all five of the occupants were soon free of the aircraft but uncomfortably close to what might, at any minute, become a catastrophic explosion.

The crew needed little urging when the F/O shouted, "Come on you lot, bloody well run". From a safe distance

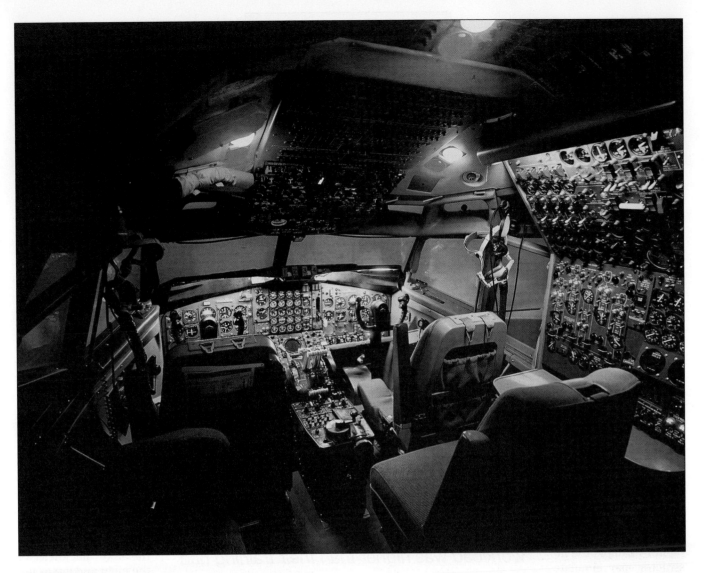

The cockpit of a 707, no doubt a busy place to be during this epic flight. The flight engineer's panel is aft of the pilots and to the right of the picture. (Boeing)

they watched the arrival of the fire crews who managed to extinguish the blaze and save the cargo – the aircraft would never fly again!

It had been just 24 minutes since they lost both engines, 24 minutes of terror and hard physical and mental work. Thanks to their experience and training and, as the F/O later commented, 'bloody good team work' – they had not only saved their own lives but the cargo as well. The Guild of Air Pilots & Navigators subsequently presented the entire crew with the Hugh Gordon Burge Memorial Award for their outstanding feat of bravery and airmanship.

Later investigation found that a fatigue failure of the engine pylon mounting had caused the number 3 engine to separate in the turbulence; the violence of the separation probably shaking off the second engine immediately thereafter.

There was a known corrosion problem in this area which had been rectified by Boeing. They had circulated advice on regular inspections of the area in question and had designed new and stronger components. The list of second line operators who had owned the aircraft in later years had probably not seen the expense of such replacements as a viable option thus placing lives at risk.

The long periods of storage exposed to the vagaries of English weather had also no doubt, accelerated the corrosion problem.

The French military pilots were amazed at the crews' prodigious efforts which were fully revealed at the two-day enquiry held at the Istres base during which Captain Bergelund apologised on behalf of the crew for 'frying' the Istres runway!

At the end of the enquiry the staff at the base held a luncheon in honour of the crew and, as they entered the room, the French pilots assembled stood as one and saluted them. During the lunch, a French pilot who flew the military tanker version of the 707, the KC-135, mentioned that in such an emergency they would have bailed out using their parachutes and asked "Why did you stay with the aeroplane?"

"Easy", said Martin, "No parachutes!"

Glossary
'Turb' mode – an operational mode of the autopilot which maintains aircraft heading and attitude only. It did not lock onto the selected altitude thus allowing the autopilot to ride severe bumps without excessive control deflection to regain the selected altitude.

CHAPTER TWELVE

A Hard Day at the Office

Flightcrews undergo rigorous and continuous training and checking. The program to train an experienced First Officer to Captain can take six months and he will already have had many years of flying experience behind him.

All crewmembers undergo searching licence renewal checks every year (some more frequently) to ensure that they have maintained the required standard. Their medical fitness is also checked, usually twice a year. There are not many professions where the licence to practice is renewed annually both for skills and health. Their job is continually on the line; high standards are demanded and must be met. It is thankfully only on very rare occasions that crews are called upon to actually exercise all these skills whilst flying an otherwise routine flight.

These days the training and checks are carried out in a simulator in which all the emergencies that can arise can be realistically reproduced and practised at a considerably lower cost and at no risk compared with flying an aircraft for the same purpose. The philosophy behind these training and checkrides is that the pilot is tested to a reasonable limit, the intention is not to 'break' the crewmember. For this reason it is not usual to simulate more than two emergencies at one time.

For example the instructor may simulate an engine fire and, when that has been actioned, simulate a problem with the undercarriage requiring further checklists and possibly an emergency or precautionary landing. Even so the workload can be extremely high and all the ramifications of each problem have to be thought out and dealt with demonstrating a high degree of proficiency.

In 'real time' flying operations and on extremely rare occasions, 'Murphy' strikes and pays little regard to the convention that two emergencies are sufficient at any one time! Such was the case on February 24th 1989 when United Flight 811 departed Honolulu bound for Sydney, Australia.

United Flight 811 was operated by the early series Boeing 747-100 series aircraft, the 'three holer' as it was called by crews, referring to the three upper deck windows which distinguished it from later models which had five or more windows upstairs. The flight was under the command of Captain David Cronin who had served 35 years with United and had 28,000 flying hours of experience under his belt. At age 59, Captain Cronin looked forward to uneventful and routine flying leading up to his retirement at the end of a long and successful career.

Combined with First Officer Gregory Slader's 14,500 hours and the 20,000 plus hours that Second Officer

Randal Thomas had to his name, they were an extremely experienced crew. All their combined experience was to be called on this day.

Carrying out the flight planning and routinely checking the maintenance log, the Captain signed the Instrument Flight Rules (IFR) clearance for what promised to be a normal trans Pacific flight to Sydney. They departed virtually on time the only slight delay was due to slow boarding of the passengers. As they completed the start up, Second Officer Thomas, who was operating as the flight engineer, checked all the indicator and warning lights on his complex panel. They all gave the correct indications for departure and he dimmed the lights to the night setting.

Lining up on the Reef Runway, the right hand of Honolulu's parallel runways, the Captain applied takeoff power and over 190,000 pounds of thrust from its four Pratt & Whitney JT9D engines accelerated the mighty Jumbo down the runway. Almost as soon as the aircraft wheels left the ground the Captain went on to the instruments for the immediate, low level noise abatement turn to the right to avoid the residential resort area of Waikiki. The turn was away from the bright lights of the beachside resort into the inky blackness of the night and it was important to be fully onto instruments for this unusual manoeuvre.

With the emergency descent, a 180° turn on instruments in a steep nose down attitude, no oxygen and now an engine shut down, the workload was higher than their training had prepared them for and it all had to be done correctly first time.

With the aircraft 'cleaned up' they accelerated to their climb speed and set course along the airway system for their first reporting point, still under the control of Honolulu radar control. The First Officer carefully scanned the weather radar as they departed and advising the Captain, they made some minor heading changes to avoid local thunderstorm activity. It was for this reason that the Captain decided to leave the seat belt sign on until they were well clear of the weather – a very fortuitous decision for some as it would eventuate.

They had just climbed through 22,000 feet on their way to the first cruising level when, on the flightdeck, the crew heard what they later described as a 'thump'. They had no time to analyse this unusual sound before there was a massive explosion. This was immediately followed by urgent blaring of the cabin pressure warning horn. It told them what they already knew; they had experienced a catastrophic explosive decompression.

The crew quickly donned their oxygen masks, the first action in a decompression, only to find that the oxygen supply had failed. The Captain was already about to commence an emergency descent but now it became a more pressing priority, as not acclimatised as mountain

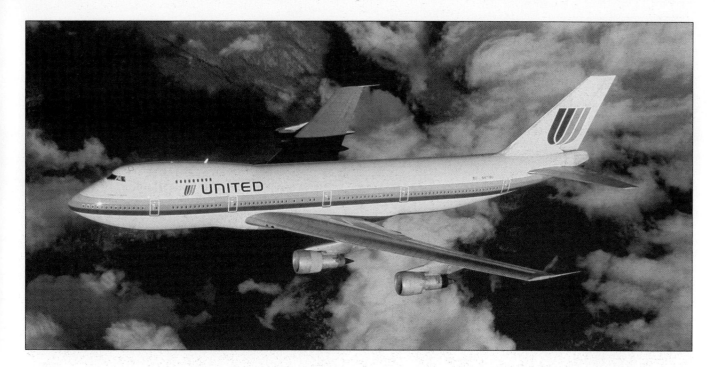

A United Airlines Boeing 747-200. (United)

climbers can become, they could not be sure of remaining conscious at this altitude for long. If their oxygen supply had failed so may the supply for the passengers and cabin crew, he had to get the aircraft to a lower altitude quickly. Complicating an already difficult situation, there was a thunderstorm ahead and the Captain had to make a turn in the high speed descent to ensure they did not enter the severe turbulence frequently associated with such clouds. The F/O radioed their plight to Honolulu declaring an emergency and switched the radar transponder to the emergency code. It was 2.20 in the morning.

The high speed descent with the speed brakes extended, causing the typical 'rumble' felt throughout the aircraft, could not mask heavy vibration which, the crew confirmed from the instruments, was coming from number three engine. It was immediately shut down. With the emergency descent, a 180° turn on instruments in a steep nose down attitude, no oxygen and now an engine shut down, the workload was higher than their training had prepared them for and it all had to be done correctly first time.

In the cabin all 15 Flight Attendants were well aware of the sudden decompression and the alarming explosion that accompanied it. The fact that a large part of the forward cabin wall had blown out may not have been immediately known by the attendants at the rear of the aircraft but the considerable noise of the slipstream would have told them that something was very wrong up front. They knew there was a major emergency and they would have to prepare for either a ditching or an emergency evacuation should they reach the safety of a runway. The immediate priority though was to ensure that they, and all the passengers, were using the oxygen masks that had fallen from their ceiling stowages. The attendants all took the nearest seat, strapped in and donned the nearest oxygen mask shouting urgent commands between breaths of oxygen (so they thought) for all the passengers to put the oxygen masks on.

The noise in the cabin was deafening; they attempted to use the aircraft megaphones to try to communicate with all the passengers but there were not sufficient megaphones on the aircraft to adequately get the message to all on board. They would just have to wait for the call from the flightdeck, when the aircraft had descended, that oxygen was no longer needed. With the passenger oxygen masks designed to mix cabin air with the oxygen flow it was not apparent to them that the passenger oxygen supply had also failed at the time of the decompression.

Some cabin crew had taken the portable crew oxygen cylinders from their stowages to ensure they stayed fully conscious when they moved about the cabin attending to the passengers. Adding to their problems they found that the masks were not plugged in to the cylinder supply and it was very difficult to attach the masks quickly in order to continue performing their vital duties. They did their best in the circumstances but it was not easy.

When the wall of the fuselage was violently torn away it took with it part of the adjacent flooring and some passenger seats. Tragically nine passengers were lost from the aircraft but the others, seated next to the gaping hole with their seat belts still fastened, remained safely on board albeit very frightened, badly buffeted by the slipstream and suffering further injuries from flying debris and the freezing cold.

The emergency descent finally brought them to an altitude where oxygen was no longer required. The flight crew had been unable to contact the cabin by the aircraft interphone so the Captain sent the Second Officer back to check the cabin to find out what had caused the decompression and to assess the damage.

He returned quickly to report to the Captain that a large section of the forward cabin wall was missing leaving passengers in that area completely exposed to the atmosphere and buffeting from the slipstream. This was the first the flightcrew knew of the severity of the problem and the added complication of massive structural

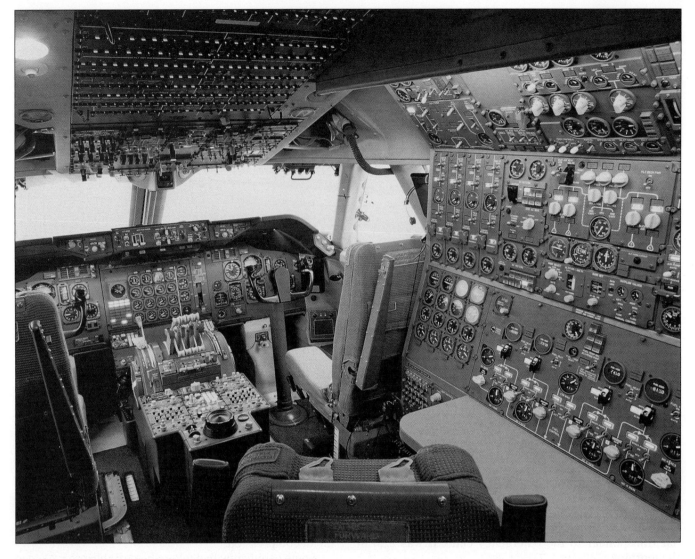

Flightdeck of the 747-200 featuring its two forward facing pilot positions and the sidepanel of the flight engineer aft of the pilots. (Boeing)

damage. There was no time to ascertain the extent of injuries to crew and passengers, it was important to get the aircraft back to a safe landing where medical aid would be available.

Now that the aircraft had been descended below 10,000 feet the flight attendants were no longer required to remain seated using oxygen. They could move freely about the cabin, using great caution near the gaping hole up front, attending to the injured, reassuring passengers and briefing them for a possible ditching. During the demonstration to the passengers of how to fit a lifejacket, one flight attendant found it almost impossible to tighten the waist straps. Passengers trying to copy their example also found it very hard. Nothing was going right.

In the cockpit, the crew could now see flashes of fire out on the right wing which confirmed the abnormal engine instrument readings for number 4 engine, it was overheating and about to fail. The Captain ordered the shutdown procedure for the engine; they were now on two engines, yet another emergency! Whilst landings with only two engines are practised during training, the practice is not combined with all the other problems that had arisen. They were experiencing multiple emergencies and each had to be carefully prioritised; one false step could put the aircraft in further danger.

It was however extremely fortunate that this disaster had occurred so soon after departure as they were still well within the range of the Honolulu radar who could provide radar steers back to the airport and relieve their abnormally high workload. They were assigned to land on the left hand runway of the two east-west runways at Honolulu airport. It was not the longer of the two runways but it was closer to the terminals and various emergency services which would be waiting for their arrival.

With the aircraft now slowed up and the deafening noise of the slipstream reduced all the emergency briefings had been completed, the cabin and passengers were prepared for their arrival. The good news was that it was to be a landing on the relative safety of a runway with rescue crews and immediate medical attention not the ditching they had all feared. The passengers were briefed on the ground evacuation procedures and use of the escape slides. They were as ready as they would be and it all now rested with the skill of the flightcrew in bringing the aircraft home.

On the flightdeck the crew was now able to concentrate on the normal checklists which are routinely carried out before each landing – but not for long! The approach on two engines calls for its own checklist and a much higher landing speed than normal. It is vital that the approach is flown very accurately since, as the last

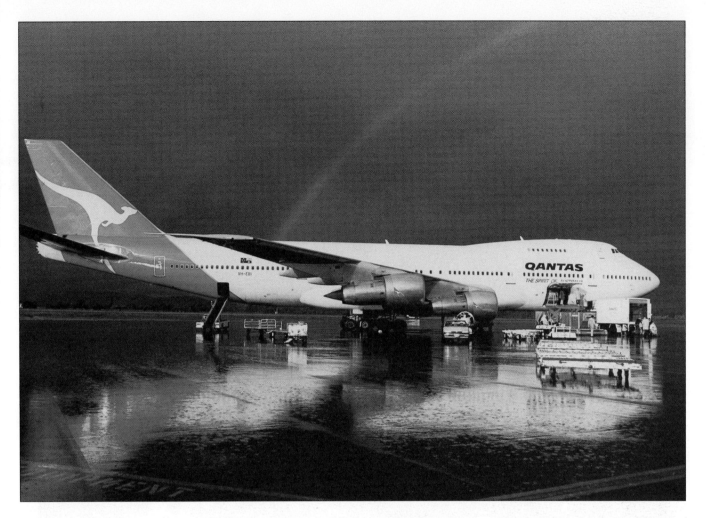

Groundcrew load a Qantas 747-200 with freight into the forward underfloor cargo compartment. It was this door which dislodged on the United 747 tearing itself and much of the cabin fuselage sidewall away in the process. (Rob Finlayson)

flaps are lowered, the higher speed tends to 'balloon' the aircraft and that can cause a landing well into the runway. With the already high speed, stopping on the runway can then be in doubt; an 'overrun' is definitely not desirable.

As they extended the flaps during the approach they noticed that they were not extending symmetrically. The indications on the flap gauge in front of them were superfluous; the Captain could feel the asymmetry as the aircraft started to roll. It was decided that they would be forced to use only partial flaps for landing, again increasing their landing speed. The outboard leading edge flaps on the right side also failed to extend. The checklist did not cover the combination of failures and establishing a safe approach speed was becoming more difficult by the minute.

After a brief discussion with his crew the Captain elected to fly the approach at the abnormally high speed of 200 knots, it was the only safe thing to do without any data for this unusual configuration of flaps. It would mean he would have to use heavy braking and the very limited asymmetric reverse thrust that could be used, to bring the aircraft to a stop on the runway. There was every chance though that tyres would blow out and wheel fires would occur but, by the time they came to a stop the fire vehicles would have surrounded the aircraft and ensure safe escape routes for passengers as they fled the aircraft down the escape slides.

At 2.34am, some 14 minutes after the decompression had occurred at 22,000 feet, the F/O informed Honolulu Tower that they had come to a stop and were commencing an emergency evacuation on the runway. Several crew and passengers received injuries from their descent down the escape slides but were probably more than grateful to be back on terra firma despite a few knocks, bruises and slide burns. Fourteen minutes of mayhem & terror with *at least seven major*, life threatening emergencies occurring and being successfully overcome were over.

It was now that the investigation of this frightening and life threatening incident started. It was rapidly established that the forward cargo door, even with its eight locking latches, had blown out and in doing so had taken away much of the fuselage and cabin floor structure.

Cabin doors on modern airliners are 'plug' doors, so called since they fit into the aircraft frame like a plug. With the pressure in the cabin being higher than outside the aircraft when it is flying, the door is thus not only locked in place physically but is further held in place by the air pressure, a double safety feature.

The cargo doors however, are not 'plug doors' but are held in place by a series of locks. It was the failure of the cargo door locking system which had eventually caused it to be blown out by the increasing pressure differential between the cargo hold – pressurised just as the passenger cabin is – and the outside atmosphere. The door had,

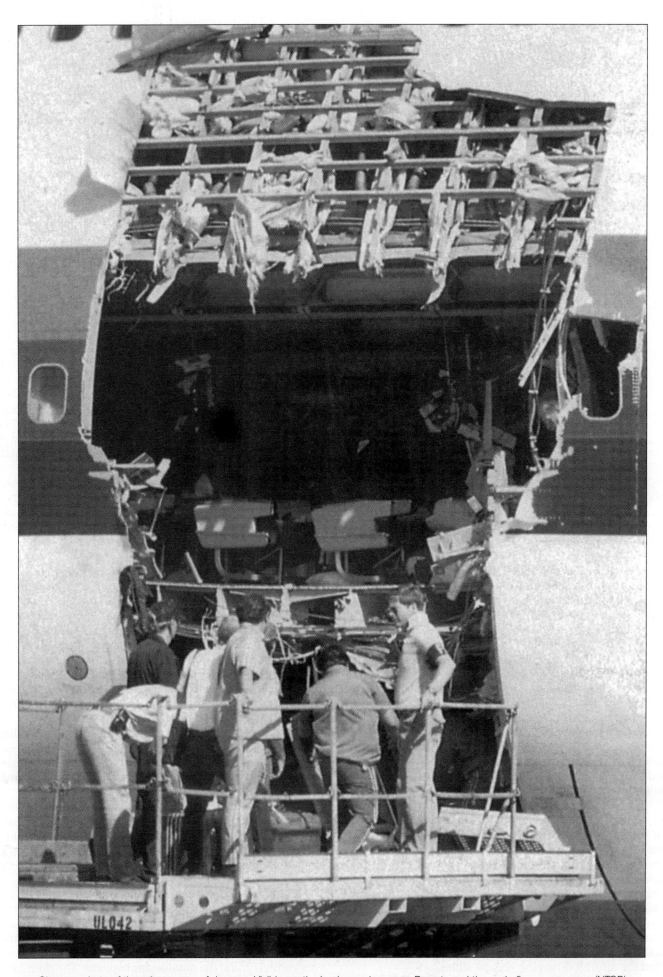

Close up photo of the primary area of damage. Visible are the business class zone B seats and the underfloor cargo area. (NTSB)

by all indications, been locked in place prior to departure, the engineer had checked the warning lights, how had this occurred? They needed to find the door to solve that conundrum.

The search for and recovery of the missing cargo door is a true life story of finding the proverbial needle in a haystack. Fortunately a naval radar installation near Honolulu tracked the debris that fell from United 811. By carefully refining the data received a probable position was determined for the 'splashdown' of the door and other wreckage. The Navy provided data on the local ocean currents. From this the most likely location on the seabed was established.

On July 22nd, five months exactly after the incident, the search was started. The Navy's side scanning sonar 'fish' Orion operating at depths of around 14,000 feet located a debris pattern on its first run. Another pass over this area located a significant target, which it was believed, was the cargo door. The site was marked with transponders to await the arrival of the recovery ship *Laney Chouest*.

In September the *Laney Chouest* sailed from Pearl Harbour with a manned, deep sea submersible vessel called the *Sea Cliff*. Four dives in the marked area produced only small pieces of debris and part of a cargo container. They persevered and the fifth dive located a large portion of the cargo door, which had been broken in two, possibly by impact with the aircraft after separation. The next dive revealed parts of the fuselage structure but bad weather delayed recovery. Finally in October the remainder of the door was located and recovered. The essential parts were now on dry land and it was decided that further expense was not justified. The search had cost $193,000 and the recovery another $250,000!

The recovery of these parts combined with the returned aircraft enabled the investigators to determine that, despite having eight locks and viewing ports for each lock to ensure that they had operated correctly and were in place, the door had simply unlocked itself before departure due to an electrical fault but no warning lights had illuminated. Modifications to the design of the locking and warning systems for the cargo door were immediately ordered, as was a new and independent warning system for the flightdeck. Changes to the door locking procedures were also made to ensure such an incident could not happen again.

The explosive nature of the door blowing out had thrown debris a considerable distance from the aircraft fuselage which had damaged both the right hand engines causing their subsequent failure. Metal, possibly from cargo containers in the hold, had impacted on the leading edge of the wing, which caused the malfunction of both the leading edge and trailing edge flaps. It had been an extremely violent decompression.

The large bottles supplying the crew and passenger oxygen systems are located in the forward cargo hold and with the loss of the cargo door; the supply lines had both been ruptured. Since the effective action was taken to prevent future losses of a cargo door it was not necessary to also re-route or strengthen the supply lines or relocate the oxygen storage bottles.

Improvements in cabin safety also resulted from the reported experiences of the flight attendants. A redesign of the lifejacket tightening straps was recommended with changes and additions to other safety equipment in the cabin which had proved inadequate or difficult to use during this incident.

Many great advances in overall aircraft safety were effected thanks to the incredible detective work in finding the door on the sea bed and to the crew successfully bringing the stricken airliner back to Honolulu against all odds. It had truly been a 'hard day at the office'!

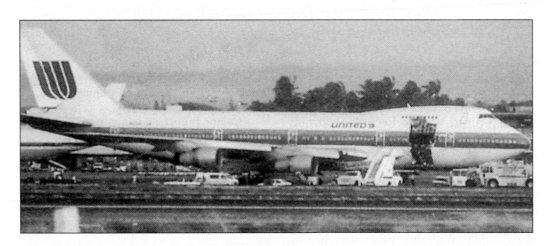

The crippled 747 the next day at Honolulu airport. The extent of the damage can be clearly seen. (Consolidated Press/AWW)

CHAPTER THIRTEEN

A Shame to Take the Money!

Pilots, and aircrew in general, enjoy their work and lifestyle so much that they are often heard to say "It's a shame to take the money" or "It's better than working". This tale of exceptional skill and airmanship may have been the time when a crew earned their lifetime salary in one day and they certainly had some work on their hands!

The McDonnell Douglas DC-10, like the Lockheed TriStar, is a widebody jet but the design weight and range of these aircraft called for only three engines. Two are mounted symmetrically on the wing and the third in the tail section of the fuselage. Since this tail mounted engine is essentially within the aircraft structure, provisions had to be made for the containment of any engine failure. The certification processes ensured that this was done.

These aircraft had been tailor made for the shorter intercontinental routes and were very efficient in the five to six hour sectors across the North American continent. It was on just such a flight that the DC-10-10 operating United Airlines flight UA 232 struck trouble.

The weather was picture perfect in Denver Colorado on July 19th 1989. UA 232 was scheduled to fly to Philadelphia, Pennsylvania via Chicago. There could hardly have been a more experienced crew. Captain Alfred Haynes had 33 years service with United Airlines and had amassed an enormous 30,000 hours of flying experience over 7000 hours being in the DC-10.

Whilst his First Officer, William Records, had only been with United just over four years, he had worked with two other airlines moving to United from Pan American. His 20,000 hours of flying experience was more than most pilots notch up in a full career. Second Officer Dudley Dvorak who was operating as flight engineer, was a fully qualified pilot with 15,000 hours of flying time. The crew knew each other well since, under the roster system employed by the airline, they had already flown six trips together. Everything indicated a smooth and pleasant trip.

The departure was normal with the F/O flying the aircraft. They received their airways clearance and were cleared for takeoff. Checking the approach was clear, the aircraft lined up on the runway and partial power was set. As soon as the engines stabilised the pilot called for takeoff power moving the thrust levers smoothly forward leaving the engineer to set the exact thrust that had been previously calculated for this departure. Keeping the aircraft straight initially by nosewheel steering, the pilot transitioned to the flight controls as the speed increased and 'flew' the aircraft along the runway centreline waiting for the non-flying pilot to call the speeds. V^1, rotate, V^2 – the aircraft lifted off and set off on its way.

They reached their planned cruising altitude of flight level 370 (37,000 feet) and set the autopilot for the cruise speed of Mach .83, almost exactly eight nautical miles a minute. Now it was just a watching brief as the autopilot navigated the aircraft on the route programmed into the computers. Nonetheless, the crew were all fully alert for autopilots and computers can misbehave.

They were just over 100km north of Des Moines, Iowa making a turn on the airway to head direct for Chicago when the calm of the flight was shattered. It was 3.15pm, just over an hour from their Denver departure. From the rear of the aircraft there was a loud explosion and the whole aircraft shook.

All the crew were immediately aware that a major problem had occurred as were the passengers. The cabin crew, promptly and professionally, had the passengers fasten their seatbelts and the meal service stopped. Whatever the problem turned out to be the first action to secure the safety of the passengers had been accomplished.

The reason for the unexpected noise was soon evident on the flightdeck. The tail mounted number two engine had failed and the engine rpm was rapidly decreasing.

They were just over 100km north of Des Moines, Iowa making a turn on the airway to head direct for Chicago when the calm of the flight was shattered. It was 3.15pm, just over an hour from their Denver departure. From the rear of the aircraft there was a loud explosion and the whole aircraft shook.

"Engine failure checklist number two" called the Captain and the engine was promptly shutdown cutting off the fuel supply.

It was as they completed the shutdown actions that S/O Dvorak noticed on the flight engineer's panel that the hydraulic quantity gauges indicated a rapid loss of hydraulic fluid for all three systems and that the pressure, not surprisingly, was falling too. It was when the aircraft failed to straighten out on the planned heading that the severity of their emergency began to become apparent. The aircraft continued to turn to the right well past the desired heading and commenced a gentle descent. F/O Records disconnected the autopilot and tried to 'hand fly' the aircraft back onto the correct heading. Alarmingly there was no response to his control input and the unwanted descending turn continued.

The Captain took over control and found that he could get no response from the aircraft either, all control surfaces had apparently locked in the position they had been in for the routine turn prior to the engine failure.

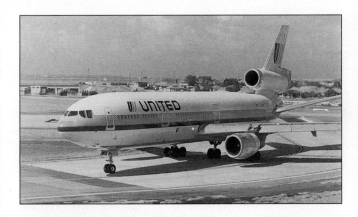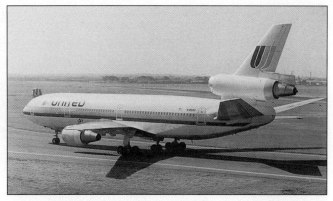

A United DC-10-30 taxies at Sydney Airport circa 1993. These photos illustrate the overall engine configuration and the effect a catastrophic disintegration of the centre tail mounted engine could have on nearby control surfaces and hydraulic lines. (Wayne Styles)

He elected to use asymmetric thrust to stop the turn and throttled back the left hand engine causing a slight yaw, which raised the right wing and stopped the turn.

The DC-10 was fitted with a ram air turbine, which could be lowered into the slipstream to provide electrical power to one of the auxiliary pumps for the number three hydraulic system. It was deployed on the Captain's command and the auxiliary hydraulic pump switched on to no avail – it too needed fluid to power up the system and it was apparent that they had lost all the hydraulic fluid and with it all normal control of the aircraft.

The aircraft took up a slow and quite gentle rolling and pitching motion. The inherent stability designed into the aircraft tends to make it fly straight and level when trimmed so any movement is partially self corrected but that correction initiates a further correction so a cycle of rolling and pitching commences and continues.

They were under the control of the Minneapolis control centre when the incident occurred. They called control and, declaring an emergency, requested headings to the nearest airport. It was not clear immediately how they were going to get there. A message was sent via the company ACARS requesting them to call the aircraft on the company radio frequency, they were going to need all the help they could get.

Minneapolis control offered them Des Moines International Airport, which was not too far distant, but the aircraft's heading was still very erratic as the crew struggled to stabilise the situation using engine power. The controller, watching the aircraft on his radar noticed that it had now turned to the northwest, away from Des Moines and suggested that Sioux City Gateway Airport, which was in the direction they were now heading, might be the easier choice for them. He commenced passing the vectors to get them safely to Sioux City.

Sioux City lies on the banks of the mighty Mississippi and has two active runways the northwesterly of the two being the longer with 9000 feet and a generous paved overrun, it was the obvious choice. He would try to get them down on runway 31. A third runway lying southwest/northeast existed but was closed.

Not wishing to prematurely alarm the passengers, but knowing that they would have all been aware that all was not well, Captain Haynes announced on the PA that they had lost number two engine and they would most likely be late arriving at Chicago. He did his job well, if there was any panic (and there was none on the flight deck) his job was to stop it going past the cockpit door!

He called for the Senior Flight Attendant, Janice Brown to report to the flightdeck, she had to be put in the picture and fully briefed as to what was required from the cabin crew. She listened to the captain as he explained the situation and returned to the cabin to quietly and efficiently brief her fellow crewmembers to prepare for a full emergency with an aircraft evacuation after touchdown.

United Airlines dispatch finally contacted the aircraft after one failed attempt and the F/E requested a patch through to the company maintenance; the chilling end to his conversation "It's a Mayday" told them all they needed to know. Maintenance came on line and, having had the situation explained to them, realised that the crew had already done all they could do. They promised to keep in touch and would inform the company's Flight Operations department of their predicament.

Finally, lady luck appeared in the form a flight attendant to tell the crew that there was an off duty company DC-10 captain travelling who had offered any help he could give. An offer too good to refuse which Captain Haynes immediately accepted telling the girl, "OK – let him come up".

Photographed shortly before crash landing at Sioux City, the damage to the crippled DC-10 can be seen on its right horizontal tailplane. (NTSB)

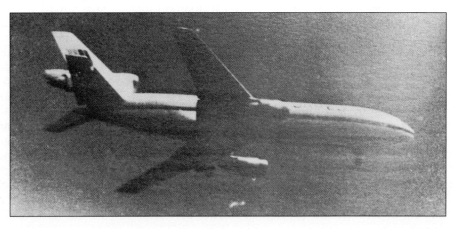

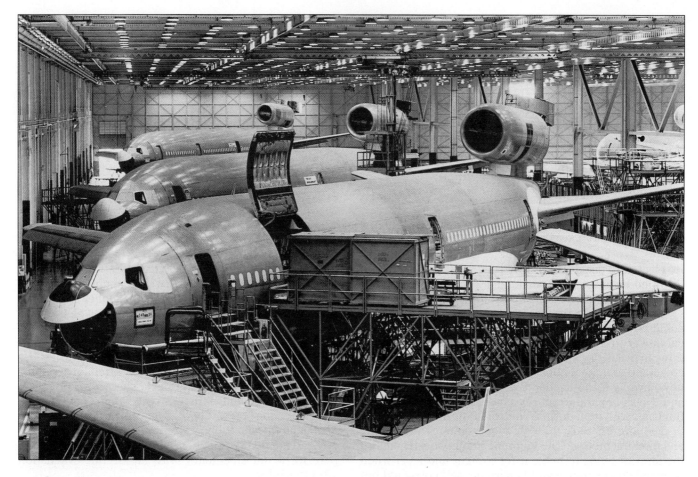

McDonnell Douglas DC-10s on the production line at the company's assembly plant at Long Beach, California. The design of the tail mounted centre engine configuration can be clearly seen in this photo. (McDonnell Douglas)

When he arrived Captain Haynes asked him to go back to the cabin and cast an expert eye over what he could see of the rear of the aircraft through the cabin windows. It would greatly assist their work to know exactly what had happened back there. Captain Dennis Fitch, their extra hand, was a check & training captain on the DC-10. He too had vast experience of airline flying and the DC-10 aircraft.

By now the hydraulic gauges confirmed that all the fluid for all three systems had been lost. Captain Fitch returned and reported that the inboard ailerons were both stuck in the up position but not damaged. He had seen no movement of the other controls. That confirmed what the crew already knew, they could not use normal controls at all.

To take some of the already high workload off him, the Captain, now flying the aircraft, asked Captain Fitch to operate the thrust levers as he called for power variations to manoeuvre the aircraft. This he did, kneeling on the flightdeck floor behind the central control console operating the two remaining engines with one thrust lever in each hand. He started by attempting to put a stop to the pitching and rolling motion that had been plaguing them. He found that, even dedicating his sole attention to this task; he could not fully arrest the movement.

As he had returned from the passenger cabin he had noted the cabin crew going calmly and quietly about their task of preparing the cabin for the emergency landing. He mentioned this to Captain Haynes to reassure

him that at least things were going well in the cabin. It would take some of the load off the captain.

Despite Captain Fitch's best efforts, the aircraft continued to make unwanted orbits to the right and continued in its descent. This did not augur well for an actual approach and landing which would require accurate directional and height control, not to mention some containment of the speed and pitch changes which would come with gear extension. Captain Haynes informed the Sioux City controller, to whom they had now been transferred, that they would have to make a forced landing. Captain Fitch, listening to this report and becoming increasingly frustrated and concerned at the minimal control he was able to achieve shouted -

"Get this thing down – we're in trouble!" The question was how?

Captain Haynes hearing this from another expert mentally committed himself to a landing at Sioux City, it was the nearest airport. The quicker they could get down the better. Obtaining the speeds for a 'no flap' landing from his First Officer and, having little time and no spare hands to thumb through the approach plate diagrams, he asked the Sioux City controller for the frequency of the instrument landing system.

That would help him assess his approach path better although he did not expect for one minute to be able to follow it accurately as on a normal approach. The controller passed back the details for runway 31, the longer of the two in use, and gave their position as only 35 miles to the northeast. They were currently heading to the north but Captain Fitch had managed to stop the continuous descending turns.

"Dump fuel down to cutoff" ordered the Captain to lighten the aircraft and minimise fire risk on landing.

"Give me a 10 to 15 degree turn to the left" he asked of Fitch trying to slowly but surely get the aircraft lined up for what would be an extended approach.

Anything more than a shallow bank could well complicate things further, better to inch up on it. The company called to say that they were seeking further advice from the engineering department and they would call again in about five minutes. Any advice that would help them was coming far too slowly, but then this was not an everyday event. He called the cabin to assure himself that all was now ready and did not promise a smooth touchdown.

It had been impossible to stop the continuous rolling and pitching motion and, if they were able to get near the runway, there was no telling exactly how or where it would land. He would pass the "brace' warning over the PA when landing was imminent which the cabin staff would be relaying loudly as they themselves took up the brace position. Emergency vehicles were all being put in readiness and would be waiting at Sioux City – it was now all up to the crew.

More information from a cabin crewmember that she had noticed damage on the tailplane prompted the engineer to momentarily leave the flightdeck to see how bad it was. Squinting through the cabin windows at the back he could make out that there was considerable damage to the leading edge of the tailplane. The engine failure had obviously been a catastrophic disintegration throwing out debris to hit the tailplane that far out. He had seen enough and returned to the flightdeck with the bad news for the Captain advising the Senior Flight Attendant on the way to make the passenger briefing "quick and dirty!" – in other words make it quick.

Having no hydraulic power remaining the crew now started the alternative landing gear extension procedure. This had to be closely monitored since the gear, having been released, freefalls into place and could cause uncontrollable trim changes. It was successful and almost immediately the company engineering department called them to say, not surprisingly, that they had no useful advice to offer. Presumably they ended with a good luck wish!

Flight Operations then called having learnt that there were crosswinds on the useable runways at Sioux City, to ask if they would consider landing at Lincoln Nebraska over 100 miles away where they also had a longer runway. With the potentially high landing speeds they saw that as a better alternative with more margin for safety. Understandably, and for whatever reason, they did not receive a reply from the aircraft!

Now well below 10,000 feet and only 21 miles from the airport by radar the action on the flightdeck began to get intense. They had one shot at a landing and had to get it right – there would be no second chance. The controller called to give them directions to keep them away from the city itself and asked them to turn onto a southerly heading. There was a high radio tower just five miles to their right which could be a hazard in their descent. Highlighting this to the crew the controller asked whether they could steepen up their turn. The Captain replied that they were trying to make a 30° bank, slightly steeper than the aircraft would normally make with full control capability.

Captain Fitch found it too much. He was having the utmost difficulty merely controlling the aircraft; a 30° bank was out of the question. The cockpit voice recorder transcript tells the story as Fitch realised he could not comply with the controller's request.
CAPTAIN FITCH: "I can't handle that steepness of bank.... Can't handle that amount of bank."
F/O: "We're going to have to try it straight ahead Al."
APPROACH: "If you can hold that altitude, your turn onto 180° will put you about 10 miles east of the airport."
CAPTAIN: "That's what we're trying to do."
F/O: "We'd better try to set up a shallow descent."
CAPTAIN: "We want to get as close to the airport as possible. Get on the air and tell them we got about four minutes to go."

As the F/O began to transmit the Captain changed his mind, thinking it more important to inform the cabin that they were imminently about to arrive. He ordered the F/O to make the PA announcement.

Captain Haynes finally had to abandon all attempts to make the left turn requested by the controller onto the southerly heading, the aircraft simply did not want to go that way but had a strong tendency to turn to the right. He decided to let it have its head and get onto that heading the other way around. Eventually they levelled out on the requested heading and reported the fact to radar control but their success was short lived. The aircraft started another swing to the right.

They managed to stop the turn after a short moment but the choice of the desirable long runway was now becoming unrealistic. Captain Haynes decided that any runway was better than no runway at all and elected to try for runway 22 which, although out of service, was clear. The airport and runway lay dead ahead 13 miles away.

The crewmembers secured their safety harnesses and stowed all loose articles in the cockpit that might cause injury in a rough landing.

"OK, we have the runway in sight and thanks for your help" radioed the Captain.

The controller gave them the current wind and cleared them for landing. The Captain made the final decision to land on the closed runway and informed the controller.

"The runway you're lined up on is runway 22 which is closed. But we'll work that sir... we're getting the equipment off the other runway, they'll line up for that one".

All that remained of the rear section of the airliner. (NTSB)

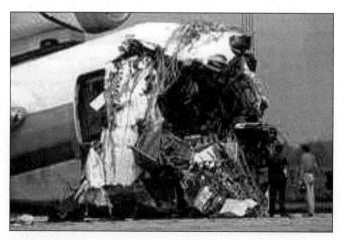

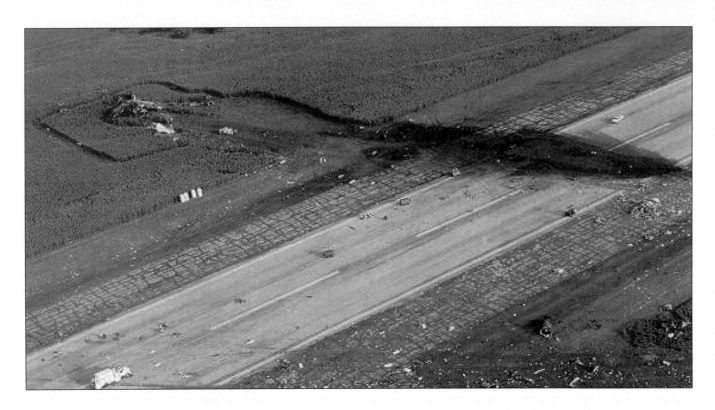

Scorch and impact marks signify the arrival of the DC-10 where it has skidded across the runway and into a cornfield. (NTSB)

The emergency vehicles rapidly repositioned themselves to the side of the chosen runway.

"How long is it?" enquired the Captain needing to know what he was up against.

"Runway 22 is 6600 feet long... but there's an open field at the far end, and the winds should present no problem" replied the controller.

Captain Fitch still knelt at the centre console desperately trying to keep the aircraft level and descending at a desirable speed. In this position he could not strap himself in, he was not only doing a fine job but also consciously risking his life for the sake of the passengers and crew. He would have to leave this position and strap into the jump seat before impact.

The shorter runway and the high, no flap landing speed made his task vitally important although an overrun into a field might present some stopping power, it would also inhibit quick access for the rescue vehicles. It was better to stop on the runway if it was humanely possible. He had never worked as hard on speed control and the combined task of having the aircraft cross the threshold at around 100 feet and aligned with the runway was superhuman. The aircraft was still oscillating in pitch causing the speed to fluctuate around 215 knots, about 15 knots higher than planned but that was acceptable in the circumstances, the rate of descent at 1600 feet per minute was far too high though, it had to be reduced.

About one minute from touchdown the F/O gave the brace order to the cabin adding,

"... for the roughest landing you've ever made!"

They were now at the most critical stage of the flight.

The last few seconds of the approach were punctuated by the strident warnings from the Ground Proximity Warning System. They were nearly at the runway threshold and were well placed at about 100 feet but the aircraft began another turn.

"Close the throttles" ordered the Captain urgently attempting to lose some of the excess speed and prepare for touchdown.

Captain Fitch now had an unanswerable dilemma.

"No – I can't pull them off or we'll lose it. That's what's turning us" He needed the power for the vital final directional control of the aircraft and to keep the wings level. The First Officer exclaimed urgently,

"We're turning"

The GPWS alarm "Sink rate... sink rate... sink rate" told them what they already knew. They were descending much to fast and the starboard wing suddenly dropped. They had, at the last moment, been in a no win situation. With or without power this was going to be at best a controlled crash. The First Officer shouted urgently,

"Left Al... Left throttle... Left throttle... Left throttle" encouraging Captain Fitch to add power on the left engine to lift the right wing in a last desperate attempt to prevent it hitting the ground. It was to no avail, the wing hit the ground just short of the runway disintegrating on impact in a flash of fire. The fuselage then rolled over onto its back and slid along off the runway for more than 1000 metres breaking up as it went. The cockpit separated and came to rest and the remainder of the cabin with the port wing mostly intact continued sliding off the runway into a corn field where the fire continued whilst the tail section also separated and stopped on the runway.

The emergency crews and controllers in the tower watched in horror. One minute a stricken aircraft had been on approach, albeit barely under control, then before their eyes, the horror of a seeming catastrophic crash had unfolded. The valiant efforts of the crew seemed to have been to no avail.

The emergency vehicles that had been waiting in position with their engines running raced towards the cornfield where the bulk of the wreckage lay. A helicopter with a medical crew on board which had been hovering overhead, prepared to touchdown and render assistance to survivors but it seemed there might be none.

To their amazement they suddenly saw dazed passengers struggling out through the more than head high corn. They set to work but, nearer the wrecked cabin they found that not all had been so lucky. Many badly battered bodies lay around parts of the fuselage that had been almost totally destroyed. The cockpit, whilst badly damaged, was still intact and the safety harnesses had done their job. Despite a severe battering and many injuries the team were able to gently extricate all four crewmembers from the wreckage.

The fire crews were gaining control of the fire in the remains of the fuselage and providing protection for survivors still climbing out from the mangled wreckage whilst others who had already escaped were now trying to find a way out through the corn. The incredible efforts of the four flightdeck crew coupled with the superb efforts of the flight attendants in preparing the cabin for the emergency landing had saved many lives.

It was simply a miracle that the aircraft had been manoeuvred so accurately with so little control that they were actually able to land at an airport were rescue teams could assist. It was unjust that their courage and professionalism did not receive a greater reward and that some passengers and one flight attendant died in the crash.

The subsequent investigation was greatly facilitated thanks to the aircraft's return and the fortuitous finding and return of engine parts which had separated and fallen from the aircraft at the time of the incident. It was immediately apparent that there had been a catastrophic disintegration of number two engine which had severed hydraulic lines and caused the total loss of hydraulic fluid.

The huge, stage one fan disc, which holds the fan blades, had shattered due to a small defect in the titanium used for its manufacture, an almost undetectable fault. Nonetheless, new and effective inspection systems were devised to prevent any repetition of such a failure.

The Hydraulic system for the DC-10 had been thought to be fail safe. It had been designed with three, independent hydraulic systems with separate fluid reservoirs. Each system could be pressurised by two separate pumps. There were two more back up pumps for the number three system. The hydraulic lines were routed independently to prevent simultaneous damage and each system independently supplied part of the aircraft flying control system. The impossible and unforeseen had occurred!

Huge developments in safety resulted from the realisation that the design was not fully fail safe yet. Many modifications in the hydraulic systems were developed which would prevent total loss of hydraulic fluid and leave sufficient control available even if a similar engine failure should occur. These changes were made mandatory by the FAA and have been automatically incorporated in the design of new aircraft.

Finally, and perhaps most importantly, a Systems Review Task Force was established to devise further means of flight control should the normal systems be totally lost. Most major aircraft and engine manufacturers including Boeing, Douglas, Airbus, General Electric, Pratt & Whitney and Rolls Royce joined the task force to solve this vital question.

Out of a partial tragedy, the safety of the airline industry had been further enhanced.

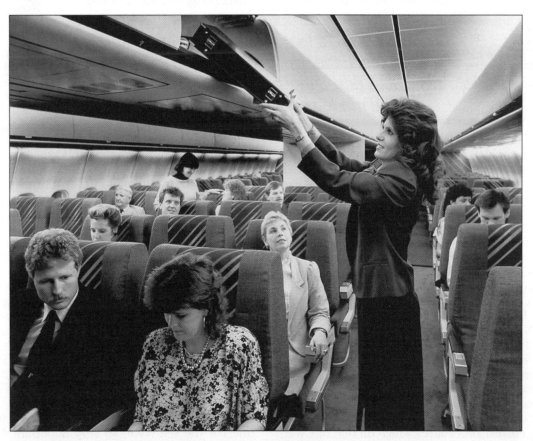

Business class cabin of a DC-10. Widebody jets, despite holding many more passengers than their narrow bodied forebears, have proven very tough in airframe terms which is something that has saved many lives where the aircraft has impacted the ground at a survivable airspeed. (McDonnell Douglas)

CHAPTER FOURTEEN

The Atlantic Bus Stop

Passenger aircraft manufacturers and airline operators place safety even above the finer points of commercial viability. It is pointless having a multi million dollar aircraft if it is not built to the most stringent safety standards and maintained and operated by well trained engineers and aircrew.

The genealogy of an airliner's safety starts on the drawing board and extends right through its service life encompassing all the personnel involved in its construction, maintenance and operation and extends to the manufacture and certification of those parts used to maintain and repair the aircraft from time to time. This gives broad scope for the entry of the bastard on the family tree of safety – human error!

The following incredible incident is a story of the triumph of human endeavour over human error with a happy ending for the pilots, crew and passengers.

In the early 1980's aviation authorities around the world formulated procedures for two engined passenger jet aircraft to undertake long overwater flights. The problem was obvious. With only two engines the aircraft had to be able to make a safe landing in a reasonable space of time in the event that one engine failed or had to be shut down.

The system was simple, the aircraft had to fly by certain routes, not necessarily the shortest, which would always place them within two hours (or as little as one hour for some aircraft types) of an aerodrome which could accommodate the aircraft. The system was given the acronym ETOPS, extended range twin engine operations. The odds of a second engine failure within that period of time were so improbable that this was assessed as a safe amount of time to fly on one engine and indeed, the regulatory authorities have been proven correct.

There has not been a case where a two-engined aircraft has encountered a double engine failure as such. The previous account of the Gimli Glider's fuel starvation causing both engines to shut down was thought to be a one off incident and unlikely to be repeated. Not so – Murphy found another way to cause total fuel starvation!

It all started in the maintenance hangars of Air Transat, a prominent Canadian charter airline, five days before the fateful flight. The engineers were changing a hydraulic pump on one of the Airbus' engines. A Rolls Royce Service Bulletin issued nearly two years earlier detailed the correct procedures which on that day were only partially applied possibly due to commercial pressure to get the aircraft quickly back on line. The very

A dangerous 'deadstick' ditching was the only alternative to attempting to land at the airport without power, a feat which had many unknown variables. Either option presented its unique difficulties and dangers, a quick decision had to be made and it had to be correct.

reason for the Service Bulletin, abrasion between the hydraulic pipes and the low pressure fuel line, had in one careless moment, been nullified and the aircraft was cleared back to passenger operations.

Departing Toronto, Canada on the evening of August 23rd 2001, the powerful and very economical Rolls Royce Trent 772-211E engines quickly took flight 236 to their cruising altitude of 39,000 feet (flight level 390) for the journey across the Atlantic to Lisbon, Portugal. Captain Robert Piche was in command of the flight which carried 291 passengers and 11 flight attendants. In the right hand seat was his First Officer Dirk de Jager; both pilots were well experienced on the A330 Airbus as they were soon to demonstrate.

All had proceeded normally until they were around four hours into the long flight. At 4.57am a routine check revealed that the fuel consumption had been higher than planned but, after checking the requirements for the remainder of the flight it was decided that they had adequate fuel remaining to proceed safely to their destination. Fortuitously the air route took them almost directly over the Azores, a tiny group of nine islands which lie 800 miles to the West of Portugal.

Now keeping a close eye on the fuel situation, at 5.25am, just 28 minutes later, it became patently clear that something was very wrong. The fuel was being used up far faster than indicated in the charts. Captain Piche decided that it was prudent to make a diversion to Lajes Airport which lay on the island of Terciera in the Azores and he obtained a clearance from Air Traffic Control to do so. There they could refuel and the ground engineers could find the reason for the apparent heavy fuel consumption.

The situation however got steadily worse. The crew could not know that a fuel pipe in one of the engines had cracked and that the extra fuel was not being consumed by the engines but was spilling out into the slipstream.

Captain Piche declared an emergency at 5.48am, just under an hour from the time the first inkling of trouble had revealed itself. He informed the controller that he was no longer sure that he could reach Lajes Airport and that there was a likelihood that he would have to ditch. The cabin attendants were informed and instructed to prepare the cabin for a water landing and brief the passengers, a prudent move which nonetheless caused great anxiety among the passengers.

Luckily daylight had dawned and the weather was fine but the sea state, so very important for a trouble free ditching, was an unknown factor. It is always important to carry out a ditching (happily an almost unheard

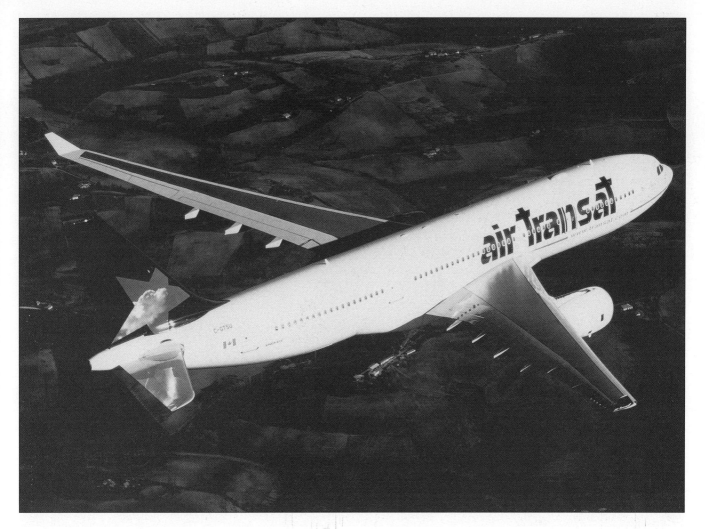

An Air Transat A330-200. Note the very large long range configured wing which by way of its high lift values was also a great aid in stretching the glide range of the stricken jetliner. (Airbus)

of emergency) while there is still engine power available giving time to assess the best landing direction and to let the aircraft gently down onto the surface of the sea. This was in Captain Piche's mind as he continually assessed the situation.

As they approached the islands, without any warning the right hand engine slowly wound down. It was 6.13am just 73 minutes since the first signs of trouble had loomed. Captain Piche applied full power to the remaining engine and started the drift down to the single engine cruise height. The fuel readout was now extremely critical but with only just over two hundred nautical miles to Lajes Airport, and most of that in the descent with the one remaining engine at idle power, they should be able to land safely. The fuel gauges though were virtually useless, they were never designed to give exact readings at these extremely low fuel levels as the aircraft was never intended to be still in the air with so little fuel. They were literally flying on a the smell of an oily rag!

Thirteen minutes after the right engine had failed with fuel starvation and now only 85 miles from the airport the left engine shut itself down, all the remaining fuel had been exhausted. The thrust from the engines at idle power in a normal descent is minimal, there is little increase in the descent rate with no power at all. They were slightly above their normal descent path and with

eight miles to go the aircraft descended through 13,000 feet – the airport was definitely in range.

A dangerous 'deadstick' ditching was the only alternative to attempting to land at the airport without power, a feat which had many unknown variables. Either option presented its unique difficulties and dangers, a quick decision had to be made and it had to be correct.

With only the ram air turbine and windmilling engines giving any hydraulic power at all, how fast would the landing gear extend and how would the slow extension affect their approach path? With no power to offset the increased drag, they could not extend the landing gear too early but then again, they could not leave it too late and only have the gear partially extended when they touched down. Everything had to be done with split second timing and all would be guesswork.

Captain Piche remembered the old aviation adage 'It's better to go off the far end of the runway slow than to land short of the runway fast'.

He decided to err on the safe side and carry a little extra height and speed which he would attempt to lose by hard braking, albeit with the emergency braking system which did not have the anti-skid protection to prevent the brakes locking up and bursting the tyres. It was the safer of the options.

He manoeuvred the aircraft into the circuit pattern keeping the runway constantly in sight continually as-

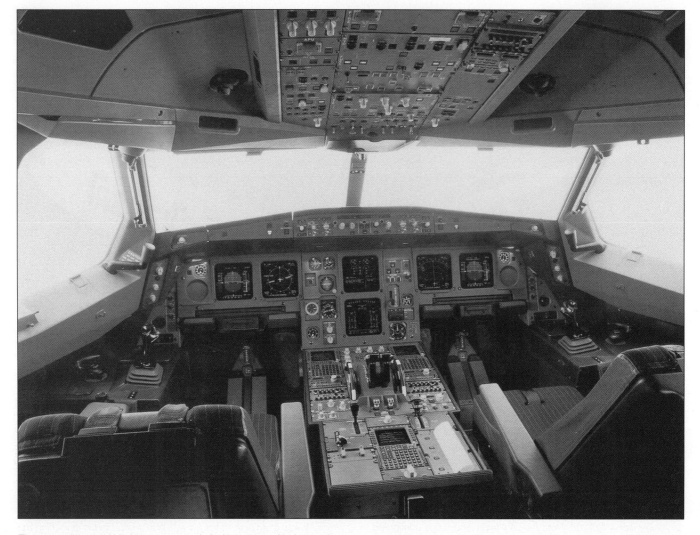

The state of the art Airbus two crew cockpit does away with the cumbersome central control column for small handgrips seen here on either side of the crew seats. (Airbus)

sessing the unfamiliar approach path. The landing gear was selected down and they waited. With little hydraulic power it took much longer than normal and they were not even sure it would fully lower and lock into place. It seemed like ages before they heard the reassuring 'clunks' and the cockpit lights indicated that it was safely down and locked.

There was also no time left to extend the flaps, using the emergency extension system the extension rate was very slow and it would detract their attention from the all important manoeuvring. Far better a fast flapless landing for which they had performance figures and practised in the simulator. They were going to reach the runway and they were going to land fast, very fast.

Captain Piche knew well that trying to finesse the landing could be fatal, jet transports use up runway very quickly if they are still 'floating'. He deliberately flew the aircraft firmly onto the ground and applied maximum braking. If the tyres burst, which they surely would, then they would be running on the wheel hubs and wheel fires were a certainty, it was the lesser of two evils and fire trucks were there to deal with that.

One by one eight of the ten tyres exploded and the undercarriage area became an inferno as the metal hubs skidded along the runway leaving great scars in the surface. Well aware that a major emergency was in progress, the fire vehicles, positioned down the runway

for the arrival, drove onto the runway and raced after the Airbus. As the aircraft came to a smoking halt they were there and pouring foam on the fires long before the first of the aircraft doors opened.

With the wheel fires under control the cabin attendants were able to open the doors safely; the escape slides deployed snapping into place as the full charge of gas broke their stowage ties. All 304 passengers and crew escaped down the slides and less than a dozen passengers experienced slight slide burns and minor injuries from the unaccustomed and precipitous departure from the aircraft down the escape chutes. The passengers were full of praise for the crew who had got them down on dry land and a runway to boot!

Interestingly this was the first occasion when a 'fly by wire' aircraft had been successfully landed 'deadstick', an exercise never practised by the pilots during their simulator refreshers.

Fly by wire means that the old system of cables running from the flying controls in the cockpit to the controls themselves had been replaced by electronic signals. In the flightdeck each pilot has a tiny control column about the size of the gear lever in a family car. The pilot operates this control column in the same way as the previous generation aircraft but the movement sends an electronic signal to the flying control to manoeuvre the aircraft as required. Many experienced airline pilots were ambivalent about the lack of direct control but provision was made for possible hydraulic and electrical problems and checklists provided for the unlikely event that either both generators or both engines failed.

A small ram air turbine (RAT) could be lowered into the slipstream which powered the aircraft electrical systems and provided limited hydraulic power to just one of the aircraft's hydraulic systems. The flight controls still functioned but operated under 'direct law' meaning there was no protection for overspeed operation or overcontrol. Using the RAT, exercises in the flight simulator had demonstrated that virtually normal control of the aircraft in flight could be maintained pending restoration of electrical power by the restart of at least one engine. The design safety factor for the new system had been put to the test and passed, literally with flying colours!

The damage to the fuel line had been caused by contact with the hydraulic line which, according to the Rolls Royce Service Bulletin should have been replaced with a

new line when the hydraulic pump was replaced. Rolls Royce immediately issued a new Service Bulletin to all operators of the Airbus A330 requiring them to visually inspect this section of the engine and the Airbus Company backed up this bulletin with an All Operators Telex (AOT) to airlines operating the Airbus advising them to carry out checks of the engines and modifications to prevent the problem occurring.

Air Transat later admitted to the mismatching of replacement parts whilst incorporating the modification. The foolhardiness of this action resulted in the company being fined $250,000 Canadian dollars by Transport Canada the national regulatory authority and having their ETOPS operations severely curtailed until improvements were made in training and maintenance standards.

This was one of the largest fines ever levied against an airline in Canada but it was small beer compared to the potential for the loss of human life and the destruction of a multi-million dollar aircraft.

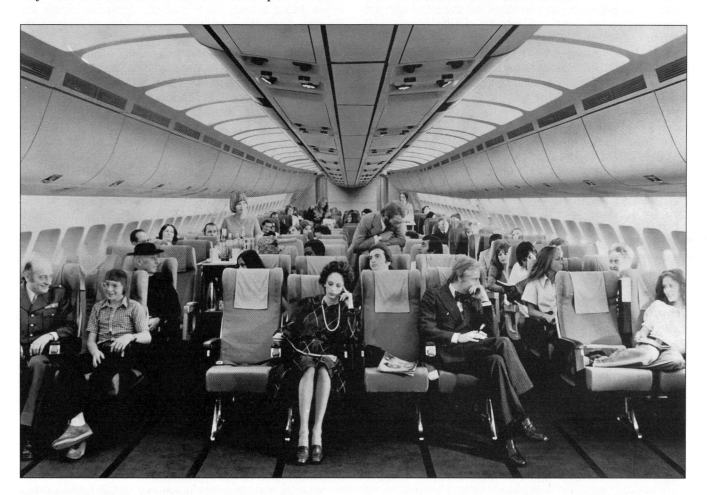

Rear economy cabin of an A300/330 series Airbus. You don't need much of an imagination to comprehend what the passengers were thinking as their powerless jetliner silently descended towards the Atlantic.

CHAPTER FIFTEEN

The Lonely Sea and the Sky

The Admiral asked the Captain of an aircraft carrier on which I was serving to explain why a boat manned by pilots under his command had carelessly collided with his 'barge', his pristine and highly polished personal boat.

The Captain signalled back presenting his apologies to the Admiral and went on to report that "The officers concerned had been advised that seamanship was not just airmanship in slow motion".

It was not only a witty reply but also very correct. There are obvious differences but there are many similarities too. Both aircraft and ships use the same unit for measuring speed, both navigate by similar means and both have Captains in command of the vessel or aircraft.

Another similarity is the universal camaraderie amongst both professions especially when one of their own is in trouble. It is a legal requirement for both aircrew and seamen that, if they have knowledge of an aircraft or ship in distress, they must give all possible aid without placing their own craft in danger. Such legal strictures though are hardly necessary as was proven yet again on December 21st 1978.

Many of the popular light aircraft in use today in the western world are manufactured in the United States. The names Piper, Beechcraft and Cessna are familiar to most private pilots, smaller commuter operators and those operating aircraft for agricultural spraying. To deliver the aircraft to their sometimes distant customers they are usually ferried to their destination.

A 'ferry flight' is less expensive and far quicker than freighting them deck cargo where, despite all weather proofing, they can suffer damage. Extra fuel tanks are fitted for the delivery flights frequently reducing space in the cockpit and the pilot supplies himself with a large quantity of sandwiches and a thermos or two for each leg of the flight, some of which can extend to 15 hours or more.

Trans oceanic ferry flights are not without risk. The task of simply staying awake for long periods with the steady drone of the engine and its soporific effect presents its own problems. Add to that the less than state of the art forecasting of wind velocity and direction at the lower altitudes at which these aircraft fly and the absence of radio beacons for long stretches of the flight to update their 'dead reckoning' navigation, ferry pilots are sometimes lucky to be within a hundred miles or so of their calculated position. Enough though to put them in range of non directional beacons (NDB's) along the way for an 'update' and again as they near their destination to home in for the final few miles. The NDB depending on its power can have a range of several hundred miles but, operating in the low frequency band, it is badly affected by thunderstorms and the signal can be distorted by other meteorological phenomena.

For all these reasons it is rarely possible for a ferry pilot to provide an accurate position in the event that he or she has to ditch leaving the frightening prospect of never being found. Such was the prospect facing Jay Prochnow on the penultimate leg of his delivery flight from California to Australia.

The flight as far as Pago Pago, his island refuelling stop in the American Samoan Islands, had been normal. He was ferrying one of two Cessna 188 crop sprayers to Australia. As planned, Prochnow and his companion had flown the flight in loose formation both navigating their own aircraft, a double check on how they were going and insurance against the possibility of one of them ditching.

Navigation had not been an easy task in the Cessna 188; being designed for crop dusting it had no need for an autopilot so it had to be hand flown all the time. Handling the charts and drawing bearings on them was done on one knee and of necessity, with one hand, or occasionally with two hands and a wary eye on the trimmed aircraft as the pilot juggled the chart and equipment. After a two day rest Prochnow and his fellow pilot planned to depart Pago Pago on the next leg of their journey to Norfolk Island, a tiny speck of land in the vast Pacific Ocean, a flight of around 1200 miles taking a good 14 hours at the slow cruising speed of the cropduster.

Norfolk Island could hardly be more isolated, the nearest alternative landing place was the island of Noumea in French Caledonia nearly 400 miles away. Auckland, on the north island of New Zealand, lay just under 600 miles away to the south southeast. Norfolk Island, however, boasted one of the more powerful NDB's in the Pacific and there were also many small islands with radio beacons that he would pass in the early part of his flight, it would be no trouble getting there.

As they made their departure from Pago Pago the first disaster struck. Prochnow's companion suffered an

He retuned the ADF to the Norfolk Island beacon and found the needle pointed in an entirely different direction to that which it did just a few minutes before. He crosschecked the frequency he had tuned and reidentified the beacon. Everything was correct but the signal it was giving him was obviously very wrong. He was now certainly lost and his only means of navigation was totally unreliable.

engine failure as the aircraft lifted off and immediately ditched in the shallow water off the end of the runway. Help was immediately at hand and he was not injured in the ditching. Prochnow turned back to land and set about replanning his now unaccompanied flight to Norfolk Island.

There was nothing for him to do now that his companion was safely rescued so he planned to depart early the following morning to give him a daylight arrival at Norfolk Island with a margin of daylight to spare if the winds proved unfavourable. With the extra ferry tanks he had an endurance at cruise power settings of a mind numbing 22 hours, a generous margin over the planned flight time which should allow for all contingencies. One unusual contingency would arise however that no careful planning could allow for.

The first light had not yet begun to dawn when Prochnow lifted his aircraft off the Pago Pago runway. Heavy with fuel, he slowly climbed to his cruise level of 8000 feet and set heading on a direct track to Norfolk Island. As each island was sighted it confirmed he was on track and he was able to assess his progress. The wind forecasts were proving good and he had no worries but as he left behind the island of Ono-I-Lau in the chain of atolls and tiny islands that form the nation of Tonga, he was faced with the loneliest part of the journey. He now had just under 700 miles of open sea in front of him. With luck and good atmospheric conditions it would not be long before he picked up the powerful Norfolk Island NDB.

All continued to go well for, after several more hours of lonely cruise, his direction finding needle already tuned to the beacon, swung around and pointed straight ahead, he was on track! Now that his flight was in the region controlled by the Auckland air traffic control authorities he called them and gave them his position and expected arrival time at Norfolk.

This was still his originally planned arrival time of 4.00pm local time, a routine call and a wise precaution as it was to transpire. Still cruising at only 8000 feet he did not expect to visually sight the island until he was less than a hour away but, with the length of the flight, it was hard not to scan the horizon sooner for the first welcome sight of his destination.

Not surprisingly he saw nothing but as his arrival time drew ever closer and no island was in view, a nagging worry began to enter his mind. With the needle of the automatic direction finder (ADF) still pointed straight ahead he must be on track. Could the winds have suddenly strengthened to put him well behind time? Whatever had happened, the island was still not in view. His arrival time came and went and he continued to fly on following the direction of the beacon shown by the ADF.

Prochnow's worry started to increase; it was now well over half an hour since he should have arrived and still no sight of land. He called air traffic control and explained the situation but there was little they could do. He tried tuning in other beacons to give him a cross fix to confirm his position but when he plotted the bearings the position they gave was not even on his chart. Something had gone horribly wrong.

He retuned the ADF to the Norfolk Island beacon and found the needle pointed in an entirely different direction to that which it did just a few minutes before. He crosschecked the frequency he had tuned and reidentified the beacon. Everything was correct but the signal it was giving him was obviously very wrong. He was now certainly lost and his only means of navigation was totally unreliable.

He called Auckland declaring an emergency and told them what little he knew. He still had fuel left for a few hours but uncomfortably little to locate an island without any outside help. The only thing that might help was that it was coincidentally the longest day of the year, December 21st, the summer solstice in the Southern Hemisphere – he still had some hours of daylight left to try and sight the island.

Prochnow considered his possible fate with little relish. Ditching in the ocean without being able to give a position would almost certainly mean that he would not be rescued, there would be tens of thousands of square miles for rescuers to search with no starting point. Fear gnawed at his stomach but with his flying experience he knew that fear could cloud his judgement, he had to keep a cool head. Little did he know that at this moment a miracle of chance was already occurring.

Over one hour after Prochnow should have made landfall Air New Zealand flight TE 103 took off from Nadi on the Fijian island of Viti Levu bound for Auckland just a quick three hour flight away. As a routine the Captain had fuelled the aircraft to land just below maximum landing weight at Auckland, taking advantage of Fiji's lower fuel costs; he had fuel for the planned flight and much to spare.

The Captain was Gordon Vette a senior and experienced DC-10 pilot who, as a hobby, had kept up his flight navigator's licence although its need had long since disappeared; most airliners these days were navigated by the computerised Inertial Navigation System. They had only just levelled off at their cruise altitude of 33,000 feet when they were called by Nadi and informed that there was a light aircraft lost in the vicinity of Norfolk Island with an apparently unserviceable ADF. They were asked to contact Auckland radio for further details and to see if they could assist.

The New Zealand air traffic control authorities had already declared a full alert and put a New Zealand Air Force Orion aircraft on standby. It was ideal for such a search with many powerful radar sets on board with their expert operators but it would be several hours before it could get to the scene.

The flight-planned route of TE 103 would take it quite some distance from the possible location of the lost Cessna but by flying there direct they would be in the area within an hour and a half. They asked Captain Vette if he could assist. With the extra fuel on board it was absolutely no problem, there was no decision to make, flight 103 changed course for Norfolk Island.

Captain Vette picked up the public address microphone and explained the situation to the passengers. They were going to be very late arriving at Auckland and he hoped that none of them had urgent appointments. It would not have changed his mind if they had; a life was clearly at stake. The announcement was greeted warmly by the passengers but it also brought an unexpected and welcome bonus.

Travelling as a passenger on the flight was an Air New Zealand First Officer, Malcolm Forsyth who also had a current flight navigator's licence. He sent a message up offering his help if it was needed. Captain Vette immediately invited him to the cockpit, they were going to need some extraordinary skills if the lost pilot was to be found in time and two heads were better than one!

As they neared the search area Captain Vette handed over control of the aircraft to First Officer Arthur Dovey. Assisted by the Flight Engineer Gordon Brooks he would handle the aircraft and communications while Captain Vette and Malcolm Forsyth planned the search.

Establishing which HF radio frequency the lost pilot was using, Captain Vette contacted the Cessna. Prochnow was greatly relieved to learn that some highly professional airmen were coming to his aid. He was now three hours overdue which, at the speed he was now flying could place him anywhere within a three to four hundred mile radius circle around Norfolk Island. The task was daunting. He told Captain Vette that he estimated he had about four hours fuel remaining, it was essential to locate the aircraft quickly and then to assist his navigation to a safe landing, not a second could be lost.

Captain Vette was keeping his passengers fully informed of the events and now, having 88 extra pairs of eyes on board he asked them to keep a sharp lookout on the sea below in the hope that at least somebody might spot the lost aircraft. The passengers took up the challenge eagerly, happy to help in this dramatic rescue attempt. Finding a suitable chart in his briefcase Captain Vette set about establishing some facts.

Firstly he got Prochnow to tune in to some other powerful radio beacons which would be within range and to pass the bearings to him. Once plotted on the charts it became very obvious that the Cessna's ADF was totally useless. It later transpired that the needle had loosened on its shaft and that this had occurred sometime earlier in the flight taking him well off the correct course for Norfolk Island. Vette called Brisbane and asked them to attempt to use their direction finding equipment on the HF radio.

Another method was to call the lost aircraft on the short range VHF radio. When they could hear each other they would at least know that they were only a couple of hundred miles from each other, it would provide a starting point. Vette had to resort to basics to get some idea of where the Cessna was in relation to his aircraft.

The bearings passed to the DC-10 by Brisbane proved to be extremely accurate and provided a good start to the search but more information was needed. Vette told Prochnow to turn towards the setting sun and fly directly towards it and pass his heading to the DC-10. He called that he was heading 274 degrees when facing the sun. Vette meanwhile had turned the DC-10 towards the sun and noted his heading.

He was then able to calculate that the Cessna was to his left but he still did not know whether the aircraft was in front or behind him and time was ebbing away. Resorting to fundamental 'rule of thumb' bush navigation Vette asked the Cessna pilot to hold out his hand at arm's length and measure how many 'fingers' the sun was above the horizon.

Prochnow called back that the cockpit was too small for such an exercise so it was agreed they would both use the same system with the hand held a foot in front of the face. The comparison of the results would tell whether the Cessna was nearer the setting sun than the DC-10 or further away.

Comparing Prochnow's estimate and his own reading Vette and using 'rule of thumb' calculations, Captain Vette worked out that the Cessna was about 200 miles away. They should be able to communicate on the much clearer VHF radio any moment.

The calculations proved correct, it was only a few minutes later that F/O Dovey triumphantly announced he could hear Prochnow on the emergency frequency, 121.5 MHz. They immediately noted the geographical co-ordinates from the DC-10's sophisticated inertial navigation systems and plotted them on the chart. The Captain had the good news passed to the passengers by his chief purser, Paul James, who took over all passenger liaison duties allowing Captain Vette to give his full attention to the final stages of the search.

If Prochnow turned the tail of his aircraft to the sun whilst Flight 103 headed towards the sun Captain Vette and Forsyth calculated they would cross each other in around 18 minutes. Also flying towards each other at a high closing rate they would save much valuable time. Prochnow turned and the aircraft started to close. The problem now was how were the crew of Flight 103 going to spot the tiny Cessna nearly five miles below them or how was he going to see them?

He encouraged the passengers to renew their efforts explaining how to focus their eyes properly. At altitude, with little except the clear blue sky and sea in view, the human eye tends to focus at only about arm's length, a phenomena known as 'empty field myopia'. To sight a distant object you have to focus on something positive, a cloud or piece of land, then quickly search before the eye resumes its short, myopic focus.

Captain Vette checked to see if the DC-10 was leaving the typical 'contrail' of airliners at high altitude. This would help the Cessna spot them but at this moment there was no contrail. They tried climbing and descending to find moister air, which would give a good contrail but with no luck. E/O Brooks suggested that, with their extra fuel, a fuel dump would provide a highly visible trail as the fuel spewed from the dump nozzles in each wing. It was certainly a good idea.

As they approached the calculated crossing time Brooks commenced the fuel dump and Captain Vette advised Prochnow to look up and watch for the distinctive white trails of fuel. They waited expectantly but, after a long pause, Prochnow called to say that he had seen nothing. Unbeknownst to Vette at the time, the Cessna had passed almost directly underneath his aircraft and the opaque upper canopy of the Cessna has prevented the desired sighting.

He set about another means of fixing the Cessna's position, albeit rough and ready, but it was all that was left. Prochnow would make continuous short calls on the radio and the crew of flight 103 would detect when they got fainter or stronger telling them whether they were getting closer or further apart. By a process of elimination they could gradually home in on the little aircraft.

This procedure, known as 'aural boxing' was bound to take a lot of time though and Prochnow was nearing the end of his endurance. He had now been airborne nearly 19 hours with no rest and he was down to his last three hours of fuel with no certainty that he actually had

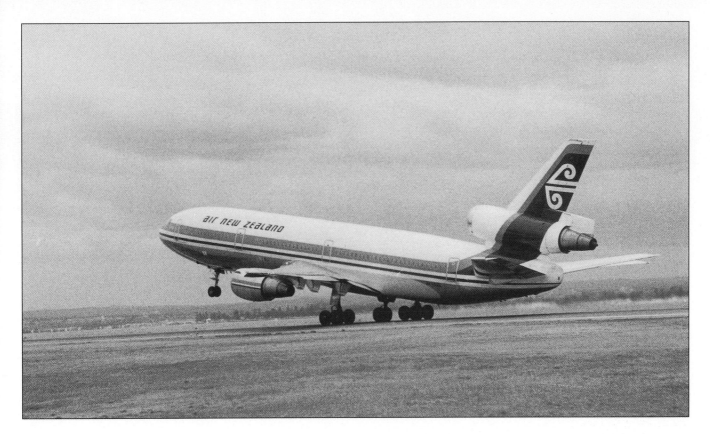

An Air New Zealand DC-30-30. (McDonnell Douglas)

a full three hours left, he was only working on rough calculations of the aircraft's consumption at the various power settings. He set about preparing for a night ditching, an extremely unpleasant prospect.

Captain Vette racked his brain; there had to be something else he could do to establish the Cessna's position with greater accuracy. It came to him. He got Prochnow to record the exact time of sunset at his height of 8000 feet. By comparing this to sunset at sea level reported by the staff at Norfolk Island and applying various corrections he calculated that the Cessna was within 290 miles of the island.

Only a trained navigator could have thought of this and carried out the calculations. Two hundred and ninety miles was just about the limit of the range the Cessna had remaining with the fuel on board, it was touch and go. Back in Auckland, realising that the situation was worsening by the minute, the Orion search aircraft had been scrambled and was on its way.

All the time Captain Vette continued with his search by the fading in and out of the radio calls advising Prochnow to maintain a steady heading which, from all their calculations so far, would at least be aiming him in the general direction of Norfolk Island. It was now dark and the sky became an even more lonely and unfriendly place for Prochnow.

It took a whole hour, one hour of Prochnow's now critically low fuel supply, to finally calculate the most likely position of the Cessna. It was plotted on the chart. Captain Vette programmed the coordinates into the INS and locked in the autopilot to take them direct to the position. He calculated the new crossing time and told Prochnow to circle and keep an eye out for the brilliant white flashing strobe lights of the DC-10, they could be seen for miles especially at night and in clear skies.

Captain Vette held high hopes that they had got the answer this time. It was not to be, the crossing time came and went and Prochnow called to say that he had seen nothing and neither had the passengers on flight 103 who were now fully taken up with their part in the desperate life saving search. It was possible that a layer of low cloud, invisible to the DC-10 in the blackness of the night, had prevented a sighting since subsequent calculations revealed that the Cessna had once more passed almost directly underneath them.

The Orion flew steadily towards the scene and Prochnow continued on the course which it was believed was heading him towards Norfolk Island and safety. Suddenly his voice erupted on the radio. He had seen a light on the surface of the sea. If it was a ship he could ditch alongside and be assured of rescue. Captain Vette told him to head straight for the light and to pass his heading but to be certain he was not flying towards a rising star, a common illusion with a light low on the horizon at night.

Prochnow was now close to the light and reported that it appeared to be on a platform with other lights. Further scrutiny revealed that it was an oilrig under tow. Vette told Prochnow to circle the rig and to flash his lights as a sign of distress meanwhile he contacted Auckland to get the current position of the oilrig, which should be readily known. Auckland came back with the welcome information that it was the oilrig *Penrod* under tow from New Zealand to Singapore and passed the current geographical position of the rig. All hope was gone, by plotting the rig's position on the chart they were surprised to see that it was nearly 600 miles to the east of Norfolk, well out of Prochnow's remaining range.

Captain Vette called Prochnow with the situation.

"If you have to ditch we'll come in and light up the

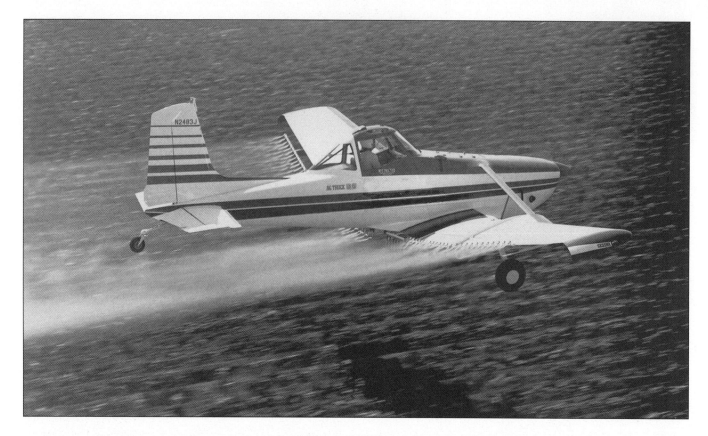

A Cessna 188 series AgTruck the same as the cropduster in our story. (Cessna)

area for you. The Orion's on the way" It was cold comfort for Prochnow but it was something.

While the Captain was speaking to Prochnow, First Officer Dovey programmed the INS with the rig's coordinates and, once again, they locked in the autopilot and the big jet turned towards the now certain position of the Cessna still circling the rig.

The crew of the rig had seen the Cessna circling with the navigation lights flashing and quickly realised that it was an aircraft in trouble. Every available light was switched on to let the pilot know that they had seen him and that they were aware of his plight. They had already launched a lifeboat which was standing by to rescue the downed pilot. Prochnow decided to descend and survey the sea condition to assess his best heading for ditching.

What he saw was ominous. There was a heavy swell running. Being an old Navy pilot he knew that landing into a swell was a recipe for disaster, he would have to make an approach while he still had the engine running landing along the swell and cushioning the touchdown with engine power. Even then the boat might not find him between the huge swell.

Flight 103 all the time was speeding towards the position of the rig where, at last, they would join up with the Cessna. With the extreme accuracy of the INS they would arrive within yards of the rig and, now that it was fully lit, see it long before. In the blackness ahead, however, they could see nothing and the Cessna's radio transmissions were beginning to fade. What could possibly have gone wrong now? Captain Vette requested the radio frequency that the rig was using so that he could check the position directly with the navigator on board. As soon as he got in touch the problem was resolved.

Auckland had inadvertently transcribed one digit in the position. Quickly plotting the new and correct position on the chart they found that the rig, and the Cessna, were much closer to Norfolk Island than they had previously thought. It was just, but only just, within range of the Cessna if Prochnow's fuel calculations were correct. Amazingly the position was also extremely close to the two positions which Vette and Forsyth had calculated by their 'rule of thumb' sightings of the sun and their radio search and cross-checked with the radio bearings from Brisbane. Captain Vette passed the good news to Prochnow and commenced a descent as they neared the rig to get a better chance of sighting the Cessna this time.

An exchange of calculations based on the estimated fuel remaining and distance to Norfolk Island convinced Captain Vette that the Cessna would just get there but the decision had to be Prochnow's. He had the option of ditching in the unfriendly sea near the rig with rescue at hand or attempt to reach Norfolk Island and take the chance of his engine quitting on the way. He made up his mind.

"I'll go for Norfolk" he told Vette.

Vette passed him a heading from the supremely accurate INS and arranged to accompany the tiny aircraft all the way, circling if their higher speed caused Prochnow to lose sight of them. Prochnow turned the tiny Cessna away from the bright and inviting lights of the rig and headed into the blackness placing his trust in the heading given to him by Captain Vette and in his own fuel calculations.

On Flight 103, up in the high visibility cockpit of the DC-10, Captain Vette and his crew finally sighted the Cessna below them. Wishing to share the happy moment with his ever patient passengers he spoke again on the PA carefully directing their eyes to the dim lights of the Cessna below them. One by one, their eyes adjusting to the dark night they spotted the aircraft and a great cheer went up.

Prochnow followed the huge jet keeping well out of the way of the lethal vortices from the wings tips, made even more violent by flying at the reduced speed. The Orion was now nearly 'on station' and Captain Vette passed that good news to the determined Prochnow and handing over the 'shepherd' duties to the Royal New Zealand Air Force for the last few nail biting miles into Norfolk Island.

Prochnow had now been in the air for over 22 hours, and his fuel should have been exhausted but while the search was going on he had reduced the power setting to give the maximum endurance. It was only the fuel that he had saved that was now keeping him in the air. Like 'extra time' at a football match everything depended on the last few minutes. The engine could stop at any moment plunging him and the aircraft into a very dangerous deadstick night ditching into a turbulent sea.

The Orion, able to fly slower than the DC-10, was now formating out on Prochnow's wing – a very comforting sight. Ahead, the slowly dimming strobe lights of Flight 103 moved across the sky as Captain Vette, knowing that he had done all that could be done finally headed his aircraft for Auckland. They still eagerly kept radio watch monitoring the progress of the Cessna and waiting anxiously to hear news of Prochnow's safe arrival.

As his airtime approached 23 hours Prochnow crossed the coast of Norfolk Island and shortly after touched down on the runway. The planned endurance of the aircraft had been 22 hours; his total time in the air was 23 hours and five minutes!

Captain Vette on the homeward bound DC-10 grabbed the PA microphone.

"The Cessna has landed! He's safe," cheers and applause drowned the rest of his announcement out.

Now safely on the ground, Prochnow called up Flight 103 while they were still in radio range to pass his sincere thanks to all the crew for their life saving efforts.

As Flight 103 headed on to Auckland Captain Vette, continuing the similarities between the seafarers and airmen, adopted an old naval tradition and 'Spliced the Mainbrace' ordering complimentary champagne for all the passengers. Of course, nothing delights an airline pilot more than a good and legal excuse to spend some company money on 'liquid' refreshments even if it is for someone else. The crew would have to wait for their celebration until they were off duty!

Air New Zealand Flight TE 103 arrived at its destination three hours and 54 minutes late with no complaints from the passengers; they too shared in the successful outcome of the search and all agreed that the delay was a very small price to pay for a human life.

In recognition of the incredible resourcefulness of Captain Gordon Vette and First Officer Forsyth the peak international aviation body, The Guild of Air Pilots & Navigators, awarded them jointly the Johnstone Memorial Trophy for "Outstanding Air Navigation".

Captain Vette was already the holder of GAPAN's Jean Batten Memorial Trophy for his dogged research into the true cause of the Erebus disaster. The aircraft manufacturer, the McDonnell Douglas Corporation, awarded certificates to the whole Flight TE 103 technical crew and F/O Forsyth for the highest standards of compassion, judgement and airmanship. The heartfelt thanks from Jay Prochnow were undoubtedly their ultimate reward.

No Smoke Without Fire

This is the story of a terrifying fire on board an aircraft in flight, Air Canada flight 797.

An uncontrollable fire on board a vessel at sea or on an aircraft in flight leaves few options. At sea the crew and passengers may be forced to take to the lifeboats and move away from the stricken vessel but in the air, if the fire cannot be quickly contained, there is only one solution, to land as soon as possible and 'evacuate' the aircraft. It is true to say though that some aircraft fires, whilst always treated by aircrew as a serious emergency, do not present a big problem.

An engine fire, for example, is quickly dealt with by cutting off the fuel and operating one or both of the engine fire extinguishers provided with the further action of increasing speed and blowing it out in the extremely unlikely event that the extinguishers do not cope. Without the obvious sign of a static propeller, passengers may not even be aware of the loss of one engine until a diversion is made.

Cargo is nowadays heavily screened by airlines and carefully loaded to prevent incompatible cargo, inflammables and oxidants for example, being loaded in close proximity to each other. Ammunition, explosives and other dangerous cargo are simply not permitted to be carried on any aircraft carrying passengers. Additionally the cargo hold has its own highly efficient detection and extinguishing system should a fire break out even after all these precautions.

In the cabin, a smouldering cigarette igniting the upholstery of a passenger seat will be readily detected and extinguished using one of the many hand held extinguishers stowed in the cabin. Toilets all have their own fire detection and warning systems to guard against the careless disposal of a cigarette butt in the rubbish bin. All the safeguards are in place to ensure total passenger safety. It is rare that an aircraft fire causes death or injury but the inhalation of the resultant smoke, if thick and acrid can, after only one breath, immediately incapacitate a passenger or crewmember.

Smoke removal in flight can be achieved by many means, not the least by the ongoing replacement of the cabin air, but also on some aircraft by other more drastic procedures which involve a descent, depressurising the cabin and actually opening two of the cabin doors in flight.

The best solution of all though is to locate the source and extinguish the fire, however, this is not always easy especially when the fire is inside the structure of the aircraft and inaccessible, the most disastrous fire aircrew can experience. In this instance they must keep calm and use all their skills and knowledge to get the aircraft on the ground as quickly as possible to evacuate the passengers safely and leave the fire fighting to expert ground crews. The crew of the Air Canada DC-9-30 operating from Houston, Texas to Montreal via Dallas-Fort Worth and Toronto were faced with just such a crisis on June 2nd 1983.

It was just before half past four in the afternoon when Air Canada Flight 797 departed Dallas with Captain Donald Cameron in command supported by his First Officer Claude Ouimet. The minimum crew of three flight attendants had just 41 passengers to look after on this part of the flight, it was a light load. Fine weather was forecast for the flight to Toronto where they would transit and then fly on to Montreal.

Settled into their cruise at 33,000 feet (FL 330) they were flying northwards over Kentucky. Just over two hours from departure the crew heard the distinct sound of circuit breakers popping on the overhead panel in the flightdeck. Circuit breakers perform the same purpose as a household fuse, protecting the electrical circuits of the aircraft from overload and the possibility of fire. They are little buttons which pop out when a short circuit or overload occurs and are designed to be reset in the event that the problem is merely a transient surge of electrical power.

Looking up at the circuit breaker panel F/O Ouimet saw that three circuit breakers had 'popped' and that they were the ones that protected the flush motor in the aft left toilet. The Captain ordered the breakers to be reset. They would not stay in and it looked as if the flush motor had seized or overheated. This is not a rare occurrence when a thoughtless passenger throws a handtowel or other bulky object into the toilet bowl. Not knowing the exact cause of the problem they decided to give the motor time to cool down and attempt a further reset in a few minutes.

A few minutes later in the cabin an alert passenger asked flight attendant Judith Davidson to identify a strange and unpleasant odour in the cabin. The flight attendant thought the smell was coming from the aft

> *The Captain agreed fully. He now knew that the emergency could not be more serious and life threatening. It had become obvious that they had a serious fire on board but could not locate its source or fight it. The whole cabin was now filling with smoke which could incapacitate in an instant and they were at 33,000 feet, at least 15 minutes from any possible landing and evacuation.*

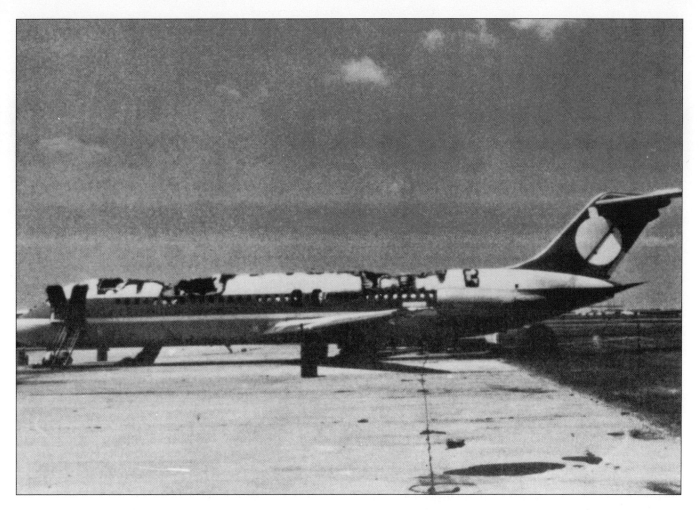

The remains of the DC-9, with its Air Canada tail logo painted out, at Greater Cincinnati Airport. (NTSB)

toilet and taking a fire extinguisher with her, she opened the toilet door. She saw that the compartment was filling with a light grey smoke but could not see any flames. Whilst checking for the source of the fire she inadvertently inhaled some smoke and shut the door momentarily while she got assistance.

The senior flight attendant, Sergio Benetti took charge and sent flight attendant Laura Kayama to inform the Captain and then to assist Davidson move passengers forward in the cabin away from the source of the smoke. Benetti then armed himself with the fire extinguisher and reopened the toilet door. He could see black smoke seeping out of the cabin walls and from behind the washbasin but still no flames. He immediately discharged the fire extinguisher into the toilet aiming the contents at what he believed to be the source of the smoke in accordance with company procedures. He then closed the toilet door to let the carbon dioxide do its work. They were all working with polished proficiency to solve the crisis.

Captain Cameron on hearing the news realised immediately that he had more than an overheated motor on his hands. Fully aware of the importance of dealing with a toilet fire quickly and efficiently he sent F/O Ouimet back to assess the situation and report back to him. Unaware of the already dense smoke in the rear of the cabin, Ouimet departed without his smoke goggles. The senior flight attendant met him mid cabin and told him of the action he had already taken adding that he did not

think that this was a fire in the rubbish bin, an all too common occurrence.

However, due to the thickening smoke Ouimet was unable to get to the toilet and returned to the cockpit to get his goggles and update the Captain on what he knew thus far. He then returned to the cabin donning his smoke goggles and reached the aft toilet to assess the situation for himself. He put a hand on the toilet door and found it was hot to the touch, a very ominous sign. It was a mystery; there was definitely a fire but no flames to indicate where the seat of the fire was. There was a reason as yet unknown to the crew.

An electrical fire, the origin of which was never determined, had started behind the toilet wall close to the flush motor. As the fire increased in strength the heat had affected the wiring of the flush motor causing the circuit breakers to pop in the cockpit. Without the information of the presence of smoke the pilots were misled as to the seriousness of the situation which did not, on the face of it, seem to call for immediate action. In the confined space, with limited oxygen, the fire only smouldered but none the less, unknown to the crew, was spreading insidiously forwards along the cavity between the cabin panelling and the outer skin of the aircraft.

Meanwhile the Captain, monitoring the situation on the flightdeck, was also confronted with indications that there was more to this emergency than met the eye. The master warning light illuminated on the panel as one of the AC and DC electrical systems failed completely.

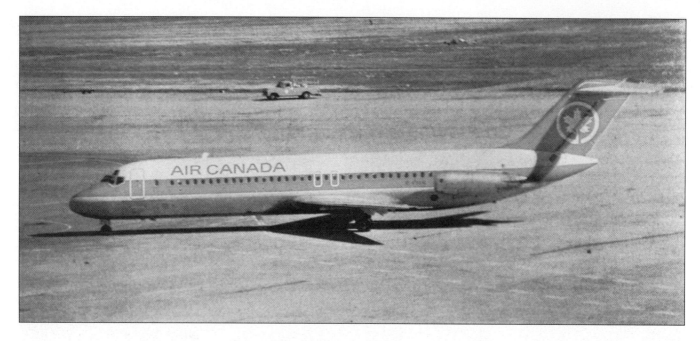

An Air Canada DC-9-30.

He called out to the attendant near the open cockpit door to recall the F/O to the flightdeck immediately. F/O Ouimet had been about to tell the cabin crew not to open the toilet door now it was confirmed that there was a fire in the compartment when he saw the frantic signals from the front of the cabin for him to return to his station. The situation that greeted him did not look good, all electrical power had now failed and they had to revert to the emergency system to power their basic instruments and the VHF radio. Strapping quickly into his seat he advised the Captain of his observations back in the cabin and added,

"I don't like what's happening, I think we'd better go down, okay?"

The Captain agreed fully. He now knew that the emergency could not be more serious and life threatening. It had become obvious that they had a serious fire on board but could not locate its source or fight it. The whole cabin was now filling with smoke which could incapacitate in an instant and they were at 33,000 feet, at least 15 minutes from any possible landing and evacuation.

If the toilet door was opened again in an attempt to fight the fire the ingress of oxygen could cause the fire to erupt in a ball of flame aggravating an already dangerous situation. Better let the dense smoke in the toilet smother the fire for the time being. They needed to get on the ground in the shortest possible time – there was every chance they would all die if there was the slightest delay in landing.

Captain Cameron ordered F/O Ouimet to put out a Mayday call, he then advised the cabin crew that they were about to commence an emergency descent and to prepare the cabin and passengers for an emergency landing and an evacuation. Disconnecting the autopilot, Captain Cameron raised the speed brakes and put the aircraft into a rapid descent, possibly another fright for the already concerned passengers since this is an unusual and to the uninitiated a dramatic manoeuvre.

The steep attitude of the aircraft and the vibration from the speed brakes are all very evident as the aircraft dives down at more that a mile a minute albeit under full control.

As they entered the descent though, events in the cabin got even worse. A sudden and unexplained noise from the back heralded a new surge of thick black and acrid smoke from the area of the toilet; the whole cabin began to fill with smoke. The flight attendants rapidly distributed wet towels to the passengers to help them

Smoke billows from the stricken jetliner following its emergency landing.

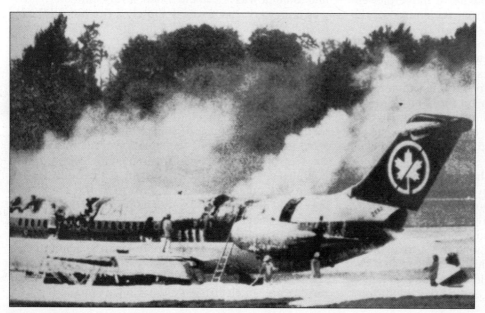

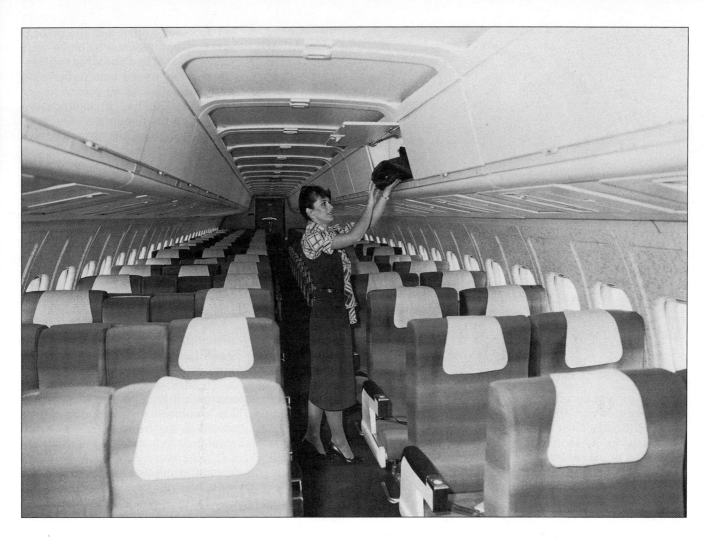

The interior of the DC-9-30 is configured in a five abreast economy arrangement with overwing emergency exits and forward and rear doors.

breath without inhaling the dangerous smoke which now was entering the cockpit as well. Both pilots donned their oxygen masks and switched to '100%' breathing pure oxygen so that none of the smoky cabin air could enter their oxygen supply which is normally diluted with cabin air.

Passengers were not able to do this since the passenger oxygen masks are designed to always allow cabin air to mix with the oxygen supply. Ouimet was still wearing his goggles and now the Captain strapped his goggles on as well, it was vital that they were not incapacitated or hindered in any way.

The Indianapolis Air Traffic Controller, to whom they had broadcast their Mayday, cleared Flight 797 down to 5000 feet preparatory to directing them under radar to a landing at Greater Cincinnati Airport, but he was now having trouble following the flight on radar. The electrical failure had disabled their transponder which would not only have given a clear 'paint' of the aircraft's position but the coded radar signal would have given the controller the information on the progress of their descent. They desperately needed the controller's assistance.

The aircraft was now descending in thick cloud and the pilots only had the one small artificial horizon available for instrument flying and this was battery powered and would not last forever! With the transponder not working they had to continuously supply the controller with the descent information so that he could guide them accurately to a landing – they must get in at their first attempt. Time consuming orbits to lose height for landing could be fatal. Finally, as they got closer, the radar picked up the stricken flight, the aircraft was far too close and far to high to land on the planned northerly runway. To minimise any delay in getting Flight 797 on the ground he changed plans and using only the faint primary radar 'paint' on his screen, he directed the flight for a landing on the westerly runway at the same time notifying the fire and rescue services of the change.

The controller cleared them to descend further to 2500 feet planning to bring them in on a 'no gyro' approach. The controller's directions on a no gyro approach would minimise their workload and be of great assistance if they had any further instrument failures until such time as the pilots broke cloud and could see the runway. Finally they were able to report that they were in VMC (Visual Meteorological Conditions) which considerably eased their workload. The controller requested details of number of 'souls on board' and their fuel load, essential for ensuring that all passengers and crew were accounted for in the rescue and for the fire fighting personnel. Ouimet called back,

"We don't have time, it's getting worse here." That dramatic reply told the controller the full tale of the crews desperate plight.

Seeing anything in the cockpit was becoming very

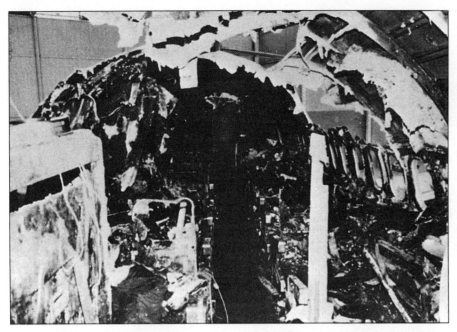

The burnt remains of the cabin looking aft from the cockpit area. (NTSB)

difficult as smoke continued to seep in despite the closed door. It was apparent to both pilots that conditions in the cabin must be much worse and life threatening. A landing as soon as possible with an immediate evacuation of the passengers was their first priority. The Captain was flying the aircraft and Ouimet, having his hands free, opened his sliding window each time the smoke in the cockpit got uncomfortably thick – desperate measures for desperate times.

All the time the situation was much worse than they ever realised. They could never have been aware that the fire was burning forwards between the cabin panelling and the outer skin of the aircraft. It was not just an out of control toilet fire as they still thought, the whole aircraft was burning but still no flames had erupted yet to give a clue as to its location or the severity of the emergency.

Trapped in the sealed cabin of the still airborne aircraft the passengers were gasping for breath and starting to choke on the smoke. Fear and panic was mounting, they did not know how long it would be before they would be landing and able to escape into fresh air. Most thought they were doomed despite the efforts of the flight attendants to reassure them, not an easy task in the circumstances.

As the aircraft was directed to turn to line it up with the runway the controller switched all the approach lights and runway lights on to full brilliance. First Officer Ouimet called to say they had the runway in sight, the tower controller simultaneously sighting the aircraft eight miles out on the approach.

"Air Canada 797, cleared to land. Emergency vehicles closed up" Ouimet acknowledged the call. They had just about two minutes to touchdown. He ordered the crew in the cabin to be seated for landing and to be prepared for an emergency evacuation. With the loss of electrical power the stabiliser trim was no longer functioning making the handling of the aircraft just that much more difficult and, as he flew the approach with this handicap, Captain Cameron had to consider his landing technique.

He had to stop the aircraft as quickly as possible to get the doors open and the passengers out and planned to brake hard once they touched down but the electrical failure meant that his anti-skid protection for braking was no longer operating. He had to balance the need for a rapid stop with the probability of blowing the aircraft's tyres and reducing the braking capabilities of the aircraft, every second counted.

They touched down and the Captain applied the brakes using full reverse thrust and extended spoilers to reduce stopping time. Despite his best efforts one by one all four main tyres burst and the aircraft came to a halt on the runway on the red-hot wheel rims. The fire and rescue vehicles followed the aircraft as it came to a stop instantly ready to assist.

As soon as the pilots had completed the vital shut down of the engines Captain Cameron ordered the evacuation and the pilots attempted to go back to the cabin to assist in the passenger evacuation but were beaten back by the heat and smoke. This, combined with the press of passengers running forward to the front exit right by the cockpit door, hindering their exit through the cabin the Captain and First Officer were forced to evacuate through the sliding cockpit windows.

The fire crews were already into action with foam being directed onto the aircraft and around the exits to ensure the safety of the passengers escaping down the slides. Three valiant attempts were made by fire crews to enter the aircraft to assist the passengers escape and to fight the fire inside the aircraft. Wearing protective suits and self contained breathing apparatus they too were beaten back by the intense heat.

The smoke in the cabin had become extremely thick and was now only a foot or so above the cabin floor. Many passengers became disorientated and were unable to find their way to the exits. Now that the doors were opened for the escape the smouldering fire was able to feed on the fresh supply of oxygen and, shortly after the evacuation had commenced, a flash fire erupted in the cabin trapping those whose escape had been slowed by the poor visibility. Tragically, after the valiant efforts of the flightcrew and the rescue crews and arriving safely on the ground, a number of passengers perished in the fire.

Despite the continuing attention of the fire fighters the aircraft kept burning for some time along the full length of the fuselage, vivid proof of how far the originally small fire had travelled and how intense it had been. Subsequent detailed investigations failed to find the cause or origins of the fire but it was determined that it had been burning for about 15 minutes before the first traces of smoke were detected. That 15 minutes without any warning to the crew meant that they were, all along, faced with an almost impossible task.

This incident and others expedited the increased and compulsory introduction of non-combustible materials for cabin fitments and smoke detectors in the toilets which, had they been fitted in those days, would have given the Air Canada crew many vital extra minutes that they so urgently needed.

Aircraft also now have 'smoke hoods' installed to enable crews to conduct close up and effective fire fighting of cabin fires. Special floor lighting is now standard in later aircraft which, in the event of lowered visibility in the cabin, directs passengers to the exits even if they are crawling on their hands and knees to avoid the smoke.

Whilst it might have been thought in 1983 that we were at the cutting edge of technology and safety, it transpired that we still had a lot to learn. The chance of a fire on commercial aircraft has been dramatically reduced in recent years but happenchance and sheer ignorance or stupidity still present a problem.

It may stretch the credulity of the reader to know that there have actually been incidents where spirit stoves, carried in the passengers' carry-on baggage, were lit up in the aircraft aisle for a quick 'brew up', there are several recorded instances of this occurring. The fire risk with pressurised stoves being used in the lower cabin pressure of an aircraft cruising at altitude, can be easily imagined. Such inflight antics are heavily discouraged!

Smoking was, until recent times, regarded as quite a normal pastime on aircraft. Not any more! In recent years almost all airlines have introduced a strict non-smoking policy in their aircraft. There is little doubt that prior to the introduction of smoking bans on aircraft it was very annoying for non-smokers who were seated adjacent to a smoking zone or, due to seating constraints, even in the smoking zone, but equally it was difficult for those who did smoke.

The boredom of a long flight without a smoke or the need to have a cigarette to calm their nerves has pro-

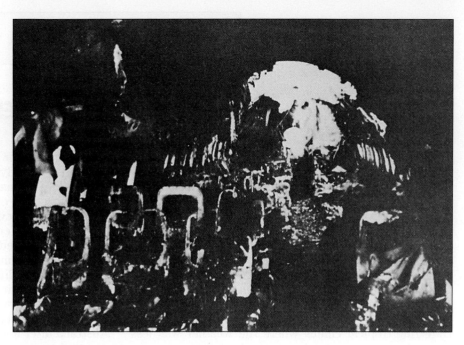

The cabin looking aft and taken halfway down the aisle as light pours through the burnt out roof section. (NTSB)

duced problems in itself with a new form of air rage – the deprived smoker who, suffering from nicotine withdrawal, can start to behave in an unpleasant of aggressive manner. With the aircraft pressurisation system changing all the air in the passenger cabin as frequently as every two to three minutes the much publicised health aspect of smoking in aircraft was perhaps not as great as it was made out to be.

However, the extremely important side benefit emanating from these bans was a quantum reduction in the risk of cabin and toilet waste bin fires. This, combined with the other technical advances ordered after this incident, have virtually eliminated the risk of undetected cabin fires and enhanced the comfort and safety of the travelling public. Great emphasis has been placed on the installation of smoke detectors for, as the old adage goes, there's no smoke without fire.

CHAPTER SEVENTEEN

The Trail Blazers

The comfort and convenience of modern jet airliners winging their way to romantic destinations would hardly have been possible if it had not have been for the early pioneers who trailblazed long distance intercontinental flying and proved it possible.

Their flights were not conducted in a comfortable seat being served endless cups of tea or coffee, with passengers in the warmth of the cabin enjoying haute cuisine and fine wines. Without fail they flew in often freezing cold encumbered by layers of clothing and leather flying jackets with earplugs to keep out the constant noise. Occasionally they had the luxury of transiting tropical climes where the weather was less severe.

With incredibly long hours at the controls without sleep (no crew rest bunks on their aircraft!), minimal aids to navigation and with communications virtually nonexistent, they made flights which were epics of human endurance and skill and, on many occasions, a liberal measure of good luck.

Charles Lindbergh's record breaking first solo trans-Atlantic flight in 1927 was just one such feat of endurance and skill. The takeoff from Roosevelt Field near New York was spectacular. Grossly overweight with the huge load of fuel, he just staggered into the air at the far end of the field and set course. Thirty three and a half hours later, with no sleep at all, he landed at Le Bourget near Paris. He managed to fly, navigate and land the aircraft by viewing the outside world through a periscope mounted in the cockpit; there was no conventional windscreen in The Spirit of St Louis. His was just one of the amazing feats of aviation of that era, the following story is another.

Charles Kingsford-Smith, an Australian aviation pioneer and adventurer, just 30 years old at the time of Lindbergh's flight, was spellbound. 'Smithy', as he affectionately became known, was as proud of his nationality as Australians were of him. Almost every one of his flights was full of drama as he continually broke records and set new benchmarks of airmanship and enterprise.

Each flight made front page news and Australians all followed his progress eagerly on the radio. There was no doubting his courage and determination, or that of those who accompanied him.

'Smithy' started his flying career in World War I when he was serving in France in the Royal Engineers but, always an adventurer, even at the early age of 20 he sought greater challenges and joined the Royal Flying Corps, quickly gaining his wings. He was soon into the thick of the battle dogfighting with the enemy over the trench lines of the Somme until he reputedly met the notorious Red Baron in his Fokker Triplane who bested him. He crash landed in friendly territory but was badly injured being shot through the foot in the aerial combat and did not return to active duties. Awarded the Military Cross for his exploits he served out the Great War instructing Royal Air Force pilots in the art of aerial warfare.

Peace was declared and Kingsford-Smith returned to Australia after a short stay in America. It was a time of great adventure in the air. Wartime aircraft, no longer required for military purposes, were going for a song enabling many entrepreneurs to undertake flights that would not have been possible without the availability of these machines tried and tested in the field of fire.

The newspapers were full of their exploits, John Alcock and Arthur Whitten-Brown achieved the first crossing of the Atlantic in a twin engined Vickers Vimy taking just under sixteen and a half hours. The Australian aviator brothers Ross and Keith Smith flew from England to Australia also in the trusty Vickers Vimy. Kingsford-Smith's enthusiasm for such adventures was fired up but trans Atlantic flights were now becoming almost common place, he had to find a new challenge and decided that to cross the Pacific Ocean from America to Australia would be a challenge worthy of his skills.

It wasn't long before further trouble struck and the port engine began to overheat and vibrate. It looked like the Old Bus had given up the ghost. The engine coughed at intervals and looked as if it would stop but then, each time, miraculously picked up again but Smithy knew the engine was not going to last long enough to get them home.

It was a huge endeavour, the Pacific Ocean covers around a third of the earth's surface and the flight would pass over vast stretches of sea aiming at tiny islands, just pin pricks in the ocean, on which he could land and refuel. Not only would such a flight be a test of the pilots' endurance but an incredible feat of navigation. History records that Smithy and Charles T P Ulm surmounted all difficulties and successfully completed the crossing from Oakland to Eagle Farm Aerodrome at Brisbane in the beloved *Southern Cross* Fokker Trimotor with only two refuelling stops in Hawaii and Fiji. They finally landed after a total of 83 hours and 11 minutes in the air. That flight today would take around 12 hours!

Whilst in The United States as part of their fund raising activities the pair twice attempted to break the world endurance record of fifty two hours and twenty two minutes but fell short each time by just a couple of hours.

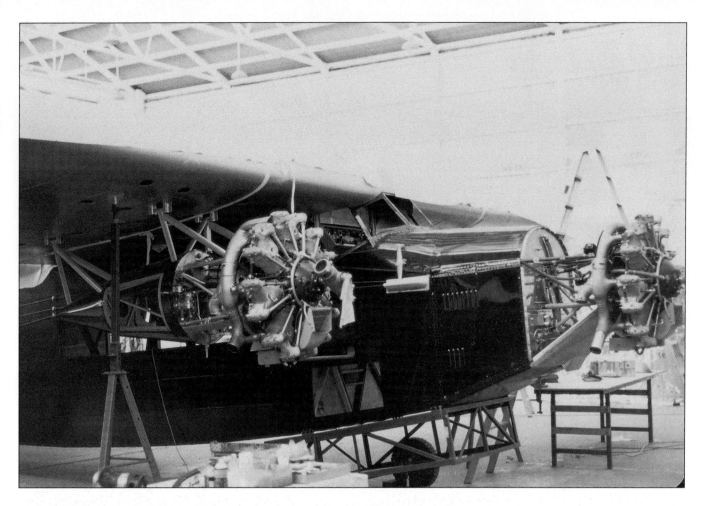

The Southern Cross *replica under construction in Adelaide, South Australia. This shot gives a good idea of the geometry involved with the wing and nose mounted engines. (A Brown)*

The *Southern Cross* later took them on the record breaking first crossing of the Tasman Sea by air but their return flight was a close run thing. Approaching Australia they ran into thick fog and despite several attempts were prevented from landing for several hours. They finally touched down with just two gallons of fuel remaining!

Smithy's next venture was to attempt a Sydney to London flight which he achieved in 16 days on his second try, the first ending with an emergency landing in a remote area of Western Australia – so remote that they were not found for a week!

In Europe the *Southern Cross* was given a lengthy overhaul in the Fokker factory in Holland before Smithy set out across the Atlantic for New York and San Francisco with a new crew. On their arrival the Old Bus had flown 50,000 miles and, combined with the trans Pacific crossing, had flown around the world, another historic first for Smithy. Most of the ensuing years were spent barnstorming and giving joyflights around the country towns of Australia, ten bob a flip and they could hardly meet the demand. Smithy's run of good fortune though, could not last forever and when it finally ran out it produced one of the most amazing feats of courage in the annals of aviation.

It was 1935 and King George V's jubilee year celebrating his 25 years on the throne. Smithy, with the enormous cost of his various flying endeavours, was always awake to any venture which would earn some much

needed cash, proposed a Jubilee Air Mail service from Australia to New Zealand. Such a flight would also establish the feasibility of a regular trans Tasman airmail and freight service.

Despite much initial prevarication by Australian government authorities, they finally agreed to sanction the flight and Smithy set about the planning. There would be two aircraft which would also carry freight on the flight across the Tasman Sea, the *Southern Cross* and *Faith in Australia* and they would fly in comfortable formation for the journey. He gathered his crew for the historic flight.

The day before departure however, a number of events convinced Smithy that only one aircraft should make the journey, his faithful *Southern Cross*. The crew were reassigned and it was to be Captain P G (Bill) Taylor, a first class pilot and navigator, who would be Smithy's copilot and would navigate the aircraft and John Stannage who would operate the radio.

On May 14th they gathered at Richmond aerodrome just to the north west of Sydney and the freight and mail was loaded and secured. The many sacks of mail included special 'first day cover' letters to the King from Australia's Governor General. They were ready for their midnight departure.

The *Southern Cross*, or the Old Bus as Smithy now called her, was coming to the end of her useful life. She had flown over 300,000 miles and, as Smithy later commented, "She was getting tired like me!" The engines too

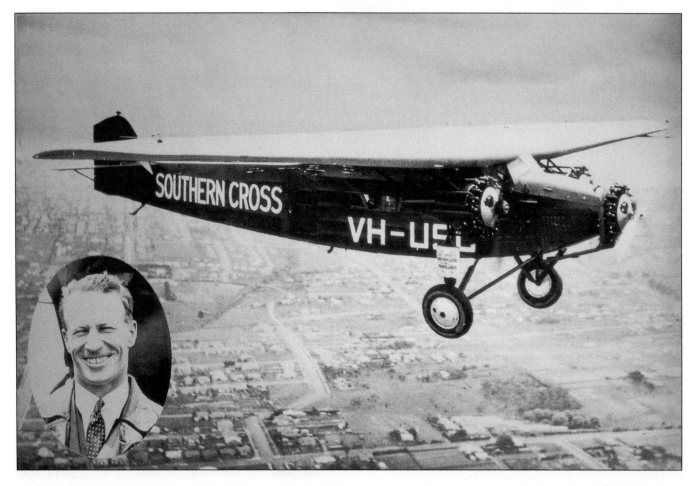

Smithy's famous 'Old Bus', one of the most famous of all pioneering aircraft, is fortunately preserved in a special display building at Brisbane Airport.

were showing their age. The starboard engine was using oil at the rate of a gallon an hour, a sure sign of old age and engine wear, and the centre engine needed last minute work done to replace the ageing manifold.

Smithy however had assured himself that, despite the oil usage, the oil capacity of the engines was sufficient for the flight and that the Old Bus was now ready to go. Stannage and Taylor had their doubts though and had it not been for their loyalty to Smithy, would probably have declined to undertake the flight. Their uneasiness was to prove to be uncannily prescient!

At quarter past midnight on the morning of May 15th Smithy started the three Wright Whirlwind engines and they took off for the long lonely flight just five minutes later. It was 'business as usual' in the cockpit of the *Southern Cross*; conversation was not possible due to the constant noise from the three engines, the crew communicated by pencilled messages which were passed amongst them pinned to a long stick.

On departure, John Stannage was receiving a constant stream of good luck messages and keeping the shore stations updated on their progress while Bill Taylor took a departure bearing and then dropped a flare to get an accurate reading of their drift. As usual they were aiming for the 'middle' of New Zealand since Smithy had decided long ago on these New Zealand flights that to attempt to navigate more accurately towards the North Island and miss it, with the minimal navigation aids at their disposal, would not be smart. When they saw the peak of Mount Egmont near the southern end of the north island rise above the horizon

they would, only then, make their final heading change to their correct landfall.

The weather was not the kindest to them and they frequently ran into patches of dark cloud but occasionally they were also graced with periods when they flew in cloudless sky but with no moon to light their way. They expected bad weather as they neared New Zealand since what little weather forecasting was available indicated that there was a depression just to the west of the coast.

In the early part of the flight their task was also complicated by having to hand-pump fuel from the main cabin tanks up to the gravity feed wing tank. At least that kept them warm for later! Nearly five hours out, Stannage reported they had travelled 410 miles and were cruising at 2000 feet but it was bumpy and very dark and cold. They welcomed the first signs of dawn breaking in the east; daylight would assist Bill Taylor to get a more accurate drift bearing to correct the 'dead reckoning' course for destination.

It was shortly after this message that Smithy scrambled back over the floor tank to the radio compartment to pass some personal messages for Stannage to send. Taylor, now alone in the right hand seat, noticed an unusual red hot spot on the new manifold centre engine. It had not been there before; they would have certainly seen it in the darkness. As he watched, to his horror, it began to get bigger. In the first light he could see that the weld on the manifold had failed and that a large crack had formed which then opened up allowing red hot exhaust gasses to blaze out.

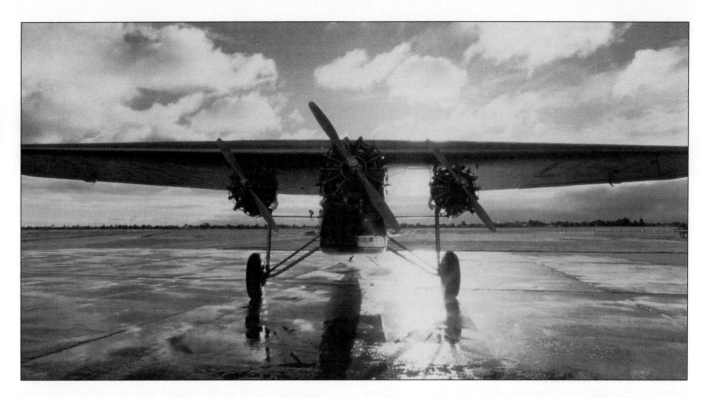

This view of the Southern Cross *replica shows the positioning of the engines relative to the cabin and some of the framework that Stannage and Taylor would have climbed out on to feed oil into the ailing engine.*

The force of the escaping gasses made it worse by the second. Smithy struggled back to the cockpit and climbed back into the left hand seat. He was not a second too soon. The red hot section of the manifold bulged out and, with a tremendous bang, broke away before their eyes; pieces of metal flew away in the slipstream. Instantaneously there was a destructive and violent vibration throughout the aircraft. The flying metal had hit the starboard propeller shattering one of the wooden blades leaving just a jagged stub with the metal leading edge of the propeller flailing wildly. Propellers are carefully balanced and with the loss of a large section of one of the blades the imbalance was causing severe vibration which would destroy the engine and most likely tear it from its mounting. This, in turn could cause failure of the wing, a worrying scenario! The centre engine fortuitously continued to run despite the damage.

The consummate airman, Smithy immediately switched off the ignition to the engine and raised the nose of the aircraft to slow up and allow the propeller, now windmilling, to stop rotating before it could cause further damage. At the same time he added full power to the two remaining engines to preserve what little height they had over the unfriendly sea.

They were six hours out from Australia and still closer to the departure point than they were to their destination. Smithy immediately turned the aircraft for home, the prospects were extremely grim. Worse still, with no rudder trim on the Fokker, Smithy had to hold the asymmetric force with his leg strength alone and it was just his bad luck that he had to use the foot that had been shot through several years before in France. The pain set in compounding his problems. Taylor was able to lend a 'helping leg' but it was still hard work and he would have to keep it up for many hours if they were going to successfully bring the Old Bus back and avoid a ditching.

The heavily laden aircraft was not maintaining altitude even with full power on the two remaining engines; they had started a slow but inexorable descent from the 3000 feet at which they had been cruising when disaster struck. Stannage, on the radio, was communicating their difficulties to both Sydney and New Zealand hoping that they might have information on ships in the vicinity.

There was only one thing for it. Smithy ordered a fuel dump letting 100 precious gallons spill into the ocean below and preserving just what he calculated they would require to get back safely. They were still losing height, he ordered freight to be dumped. The Old Bus was still going down. It looked like a ditching about as far as they could be from any help and with little hope of rescue.

Smithy had long ago planned, in the event of a ditching, that they would detach a section of the wing once in the water which would hopefully act as a liferaft whilst they awaited rescue – a desperate measure and a forlorn hope! Stannage radioed to shore that they would try to save the precious mail and asked for a clearance from the postal authorities to dump it if necessary. This message was probably superfluous; Smithy would have undoubtedly sacrificed the mail come what may to avoid endangering the lives of his crew.

The message came through that they had authority to dump the mail but Smithy, ever hopeful of salvaging the situation, did not give the order hoping that as they descended the aircraft would finally maintain height. Desperation was setting in. To reduce the still threatening vibration Taylor tried to even up the propeller blades on the dead engine reaching out from the cockpit window with a small hacksaw as Smithy slowed the aircraft to bring the propeller blades just within his reach, but to no avail. Each time as he started to cut, the blades moved away from him. Smithy's indomitable spirit concealed his dread of 'going in' with the very evident possibility of a lonely death by drowning.

A smile and a knowing wink to his crewmembers kept their spirits up – just. Finally, the drastic attempts to lighten the aircraft had their effect and Smithy was able to arrest the descent and cruise with the engines just off their full power setting, but at what price? The two remaining engines could not take this punishment for too long and they were still a long way from home now battling an unwelcome stiff nor-wester.

It wasn't long before further trouble struck and the port engine began to overheat and vibrate. It looked like the Old Bus had given up the ghost. The engine coughed at intervals and looked as if it would stop but then, each time, miraculously picked up again but Smithy knew the engine was not going to last long enough to get them home. Stannage radioed the news that they would almost certainly ditch and optimistically asked for any help that could be sent. The sea was looking very choppy with waves being driven by the increasing wind strength. Even if they managed a successful ditching the chances of surviving long in the chilly waters were not good.

For five hours Smithy had nursed the Old Bus towards Australia and they were still 300 miles away. He found it impossible to continue using his bad leg to keep the aircraft straight, his strength was drained so Smithy relinquished control of the aircraft to Taylor to take a much needed rest.

The strain on the engines was also beginning to take its toll; the port engine was obviously consuming oil very fast. The remaining oil was not enough to get them home and, without oil the engine would simply seize. With only one engine left running a ditching no longer would be a possibility, it would be certain and soon. Even the ever optimistic Smithy could not conceal his concern.

Alongside Stannage in the radio cabin taking his rest he shouted, "Looks like we've collected it this time old son. The port motor won't last another hour." He set about gathering together some tools to construct his 'wing life raft' once they were in the water and sealed vents in the cabin with old rags to give the best flotation time while they sawed off the section of wing. On departure from Richmond Stannage had been given a small bottle of whisky labelled "Radio Operator's Moaning Fluid' alluding to the tradition that radio operators were never happy with their lot and always complaining about atmospheric conditions or the quality of reception.

Smithy decided it was time to use it and they raised their glasses to each other in a toast to good fortune. All three were inveterate smokers but with the enormous amount of highly volatile fuel on board and tanks right there in the cabin, smoking was never permitted. At this moment in time it didn't seem to matter any more and, like the condemned men they thought they were, they all had a welcome cigarette to complement the Scotch.

The oil pressure on the port engine had now dropped to a dangerously low level. It was ironic that the starboard engine, known to be using oil but now shut down, still had plenty of oil remaining; it was of little use in the dead engine! Smithy, having had his break was now back at the controls when Stannage and Taylor had the same thought. If they could get the oil out of the dead engine and transfer it to the ailing port engine it could keep them going long enough to stay dry!

Smithy thought it impossible and certain death for anyone attempting the midair transfer and entreated them not to even think about it. Ignoring Smithy's advice Stannage secured himself to the aircraft with some twine from the mail sacks and opened the window to climb out on the spar to reach the starboard engine. The windblast threw him back; no matter how hard he tried he could not climb out.

Taylor, seeing the unsuccessful efforts of his valiant colleague decided that, being bigger and possibly stronger, he could succeed where Stannage had failed. Taking off his boots to give him better purchase once outside and securing himself with the thin twine, he climbed out. Using the slipstream to his advantage he allowed it to pinion him against the wing and, letting go of his grasp on the cabin wall, started to edge his way along the spar to the engine.

'One arm for the King and one for yourself', the watchword of seamen working in the rigging of the clipper ships, now entered the field of aviation. With his spare hand Taylor wrenched at the engine panel under which lay the oil drain plug. It came away and was whipped from his hands to fall to the sea below, there was the drain plug but he had not brought a wrench to undo it.

Stannage, still in the cabin was ahead of him and passed a spanner, one of the few things that had not been jettisoned. To Taylor's immense relief the plug undid easily.

Again the trusty Stannage in the cabin came to his aid. He had located a small 'lunchbox' suitcase and a thermos flask. He had smashed the glass in the thermos and passed the metal outer container to Taylor who managed to anchor himself to the wing strut by his legs allowing him to undo the oil plug by hand and hold the thermos under the drain to gather the oil. As the oil drained the slipstream carried most of it away and only by holding the thermos mouth hard against the drain hole was he able to gather any oil.

Reinserting the plug he passed the thermos back to Stannage but the slipstream again thwarted him sucking more oil out of the open mouth of the thermos. Stannage poured the remaining oil into his 'storage tank', the empty suitcase. One half of this incredible transfer had been completed with partial success; it was now a question of whether the vital oil could be got to the other engine.

Taylor was now wet, cold, exhausted and covered in oil, not a good recipe for the dangerous climb out onto the other wing. He climbed gingerly back into the cabin and fell to the floor for a necessary rest.

There are varying accounts of what exactly happened next. Most attribute all the action to Taylor but according to one account Smithy, seeing Taylor's exhaustion, moved over to the right hand seat and indicated to him that he should take the left hand seat to rest and recover his strength. Stannage then took off his boots and climbed out onto the spar holding the thermos tightly in his free hand. The right engine being shut down, Taylor had only had to fight against the slipstream on the first foray out onto the starboard wing; it was different kettle of fish on the left wing with the motor running at near full power and the added strength of the propeller wash.

Stannage was flattened against the fuselage and couldn't move. He later allowed in his memoirs that,

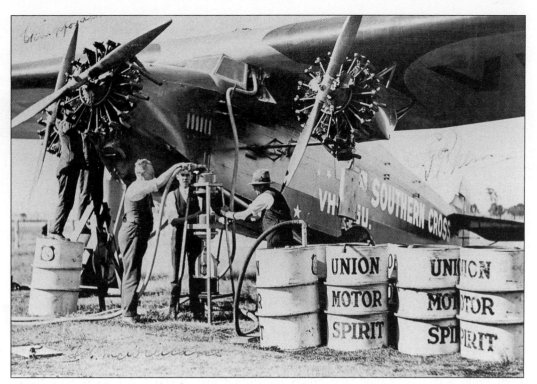

Fuel is hand pumped into the Fokker Southern Cross *prior to another record breaking flight.*

even if he had been able to move, he doubted that he would have had the courage to carry it through – a hidden tribute to Taylor's heroism. He climbed back into the cabin beaten by the elements. Smithy did not mention this part of the action in his account of the flight in his book My Flying Years, probably because, ever the gentleman, he did not want to be seen to be belittling his fellow aviator.

Smithy had watched events out of the corner of his eye and realised that both men had put their own lives at great risk to save the day. They had proved it was possible, there had to be a better and safer way to achieve the vital transfer. The problem was obviously the combined windblast from the aircraft's slipstream and the propeller's wake. What if he slowed to aircraft to its minimum safe speed and throttled back the port engine?

The aircraft would descend but perhaps there would be enough time for one of them to climb out and pour the salvaged oil into the port engine before he would be forced to add power again to climb away from the sea. Taylor braced himself for his second sortie out onto the port wingspar. As he was ready he signalled Smithy who throttled back on the port engine. Taylor climbed out onto the spar, already slippery with oil streaks from the engine, and reached the engine. Stannage stretching to full reach passed the thermos to him and although still losing some oil to the slipstream, Taylor cupped his spare hand around the filler cap and poured it in.

The Old Bus was now skimming the waves and as Taylor made his cautious way back along the spar Smithy had to add full power once again. Just half a thermos of oil had an immediate and startling effect. Smithy bellowed back to Stannage that they had oil pressure again and Stannage, jubilant, thrust out both arms with his thumbs up indicating to Taylor, still on his way back, that they had met with success.

Taylor, now safely back in the cabin, was euphoric. Stannage radioed a brief account of Taylor's courageous actions to Sydney. The press, knowing that Smithy and

the *Southern Cross* were in grave danger from earlier radio messages, went berserk. New editions were rushed to the presses and billboards around the country proclaimed this amazing act of courage.

They flew on, the miles towards Australia slowly unwinding, far too slowly! The power of just two tired motors simply not enough to give them their normal cruising speed especially as Smithy nursed them as best he could slightly off their maximum power setting. They still had just under 200 miles to safety and the port engine was still using oil at an alarming rate but now the centre engine was faltering and getting low on oil.

To remedy that was an impossibility, there was simply no way to gain access to it but there was no doubt that Taylor would have to repeat his performance several times if they were to keep the port motor from seizing. Six times in all he successfully made the perilous journey out onto the starboard wing carrying the empty thermos and guarding its precious contents on the way back only to climb out again onto the port wing to replenish the ailing engine. The banging the thermos had received to get rid of its glass vacuum interior and increase its capacity took its toll, the metal casing finally split down the seam. The ever resourceful Stannage tore up a shirt and bound it around the canister with his tie, it was a rough and ready repair but it worked.

The continuous climbing and descending was also not helping, each time they climbed back to a lower cruise altitude giving Taylor less and less time to achieve the transfer. After the second transfer Smithy reluctantly ordered some of the heavy mail bags to be thrown overboard, it was a last ditch effort and it gave them some breathing space. It later transpired that the bags that had been jettisoned contained the letters to King George V.

The world was now listening to the progress of the *Southern Cross* battling to make it back to Australia. In London, the Australian Prime Minister Joseph Lyons had ordered constant reports although it was now the dead of night and in Australia the population was glued to

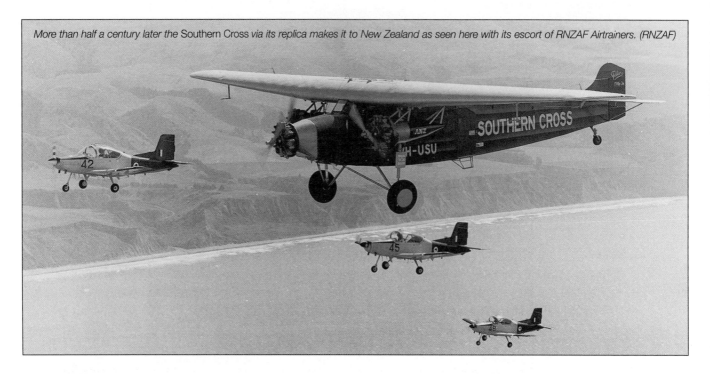
More than half a century later the Southern Cross via its replica makes it to New Zealand as seen here with its escort of RNZAF Airtrainers. (RNZAF)

their radio sets – they flew with Smithy and his crew willing them home safely. Smithy's wife Mary, concerned at what the stress of this prolonged emergency might do to her husband's health called his GP and asked him to go with her to meet the aircraft on arrival.

As they got closer to the coast Smithy's hopes rose, even if they ditched 100 miles out the Air Force had 'planes with that range who could drop a raft and direct rescue ships to them. He tried to persuade Taylor that another transfer would not be necessary but, understandably, Taylor was determined that having risked his life five times to save the aircraft, one more trip was very much worth the while. Out he went again to put the final load of oil into the port engine. By now his appearance had to be seen to be believed – his clothing, face and hands blackened and reeking from the oil whipped out of the thermos and spilled during the transfers.

Nearly nine hours after they had lost the starboard engine with its shattered propeller they finally crossed the coast of Australia just to the south of Botany Bay and, at four o'clock in the afternoon they touched down at Mascot aerodrome. They had been airborne just under 16 hours, the last nine of them all the time facing a watery grave.

The crowds rushed to meet the battered and begrimed aircraft and crew. The door opened and Smithy and his crew appeared. Smithy was drained and understandably looked and acted like a zombie, his normal ebullient self totally gone. He had no word for anyone but was gently led away by his wife and the doctor to the comfort of a warm bath and long rest.

Both Bill Taylor, covered in oil and looking like an escapee from the Black & White Minstrel show, and John Stannage had little to say. They were desperate to clean up and have a well earned rest. Their exhausted appearance spoke volumes for them. They had just taken part in what must stand as one of the most amazing feats ever recorded in the annals of aviation.

Smithy took a day or two to recover and, embarrassed that he had had to dump most of the mail, insisted on taking the remaining mailbags to New Zealand the next day in the other aircraft. Happily wiser council prevailed. He knew though that it was the end of his beloved *Southern Cross* and he negotiated that the government buy the aircraft and put her on permanent display with the added condition, being so precious to him and Australia, that she never fly again. Captain P G Taylor was awarded the George Cross by the King in recognition of his heroism in saving the crew and aircraft.

Despite the national acclaim Smithy and his crew had their detractors who claimed that the event never actually took place but that it was a prearranged publicity stunt to raise money for the ever cash strapped Smithy. The rumours lingered on and, in 1985, when a full scale mock up was built for a television series and attempts were made to re-enact this flight on the ground, it was found that with a huge fan generating wind blast to simulate the slipstream, the actors could not transfer any oil at all, it was all lost in the wind.

Noted experts argued for Smithy and his crew, especially Bruce Cowan, their second engineer who had worked on the engines before and after the flight; he confirmed that less than two gallons of oil remained in the starboard engine when, due to its early shutdown there should have been considerably more; where had it all gone if it had not been transferred? Bruce even visited Smithy's widow in Queensland and saw, with his own eyes, the famous thermos still with the rags from the shirt around it and secured by a tie.

Another highly credible expert, Bill Booth with over 28,000 hours of airline flying to his credit, actually produced proof positive. When the *Southern Cross* was under maintenance by the Royal Australian Air Force in 1945 they had found slivers of thermos vacuum flask glass and Bill Booth had obtained one piece and kept it as a souvenir all those years. The detractors were silenced once and for all and Sir Charles Kingsford Smith, Captain P G (Bill) Taylor and John Stannage were finally recognised by all as the heroes they actually were.

These were the men who blazed the trails, opened up the skies and shrank the world to what it is today. They defeated the tyranny of distance.

POSTSCRIPT

This book was not written to terrify would be airline travellers, exactly the reverse. It was written to illustrate the continuing great advances in air safety and the quality of the men and women who crew those aircraft and the simple fact that, flying on an airline is one of the safest occupations that you can undertake. There are also many things that a traveller can do to enhance the safety of their planned flight, more on that later, but first a few words of advice illustrated by a short anecdote.

A traditional 'Little Old Lady' had bought a ticket for a flight but, never having flown before and having read many reports of bombs on aircraft, was at the check-in counter deliberating whether or not she would travel after all.

"I'm very worried about all these reports of bombs on aircraft" she told the check-in clerk. "I think I will cancel my flight"

"No, don't do that madam. It's very safe you know. There is only a one in a hundred million chance of a bomb being on the aircraft that you are on"

"I'm not sure that I am happy about that," said the little old lady still thinking of cancelling her flight.

"Well madam, if you bring your own bomb the odds of having two bombs on the same aircraft treble. Surely that's safe enough for you!"

The story doesn't record whether our little old lady travelled or not but the odds are correct. An acceptable 'risk' in aviation is recognised as a chance of one in 10^{-7} or, put more simply, one in 100,000,000 times. In other terms you would have to fly every day for 1141 years, or continuously for over 16 average lifespans, before you fell victim to a serious incident in the air.

To further improve the odds, if you're like the little old lady, always fly with reputable airlines. Bucket shop 'specials' are not always the bargains they appear to be. At worst, if there is a significant delay, a reputable airline will accommodate and feed you until you finally depart whereas others will leave you in the terminal without even a voucher for dinner, at best you will arrive at your destination safely and on time.

Many nationalities have an ethos where a captain of an aircraft, or any other person in authority, cannot be questioned, but is blindly obeyed. You must be the judge of the nationalities concerned. This is not a good situation in the cockpit of an aeroplane where the duty of other crewmembers is to monitor and advise. Most airlines today teach, indeed insist on, junior crewmembers speaking up when they have any doubts and the captain listening to their concerns. The same nations tend to have endemic corruption which permits pilots with 'connections' to gain employment and command when otherwise they would not have done so. Of that I have personal knowledge.

Avoid the airlines of countries where political unrest leaves them vulnerable to terrorist activities. Even the best security measures will not prevent the determined saboteur or hijacker. It goes without saying that you should not consider flying into areas where political unrest is currently rife.

If, on boarding, you observe that security precautions are lax or non-existent, give serious consideration to not travelling. With the major national airlines of developed countries this is not a worry since much security work is low key but very efficient. NEVER carry anything for anybody you do not personally know well and, should you agree to carry a package for a close friend, ask and see what it is. You will then be able to answer the security questions at the check in desk honestly and accurately

Lastly I would recommend that 'Inaugural Flights' be avoided. There is an unhealthy predominance of incidents occurring on such flights for whatever reason.

The airlines, crews and regulatory authorities have done their bit, you too can help. Safe Flying!

GLOSSARY

ACARS Aircraft communications and reporting system. A datalink system to automatically communicate flight data, performance data and routine aircraft reports and messages. Uses VHF radio or satellite links to communicate data. Pilots receive a printout of answers to messages or a screen message.

Active volcano Any volcano which has erupted within the previous 600 years is regarded as active.

Ailerons Situated on the trailing edge of the wing they are used to bank or roll the aircraft.

Aircraft Oxygen Required by law to be used by crew if cabin pressurisation is lost until the aircraft can be descended to a safe height. Separate systems are provided for crew and passengers.

Airways Air routes designated by radio beacons or geographical coordinates.

Asymetric Flight When a multi engined aircraft is flying with an engine or engines on one side failed or shut down.

Batsman The flight deck officer on an aircraft carrier who guided aircraft to a landing by means of two paddles or bats signalling alignment and whether high or low on the approach. Now replaced by the mirror landing system.

Bolter A naval term when an aircraft misses all the arrester wires when landing on an aircraft carrier. With the high engine power settings for the approach, the pilot merely increases to full power and flies off the front of the deck for another approach.

Circuit breaker A small button like fuse which pops out when an electrical circuit detects an overload.

Elevators Control surfaces on the rear of the tailplane used to control the nose attitude of the aircraft and to climb or descend.

E/O Engineer Officer or flight engineer.

Engine numbers For ease of identification engines are numbered from left to right sequentially facing forward. The left hand outboard engine being number 1 engine.

Fin Also known as vertical stabiliser – provides directional stability to the aircraft.

Flaps Situated on the trailing edge of the wing they are lowered for take off and landing to reduce stalling speed to allow lower and safer speeds for arrival and departure. Retracted for cruise. On larger aircraft flaps are augmented by the electric stabiliser to counter large changes of centre of gravity.

F/O First Officer or deputy Captain.

Flight Level Altitudes determined by a 'standard' altimeter setting 1013.2 millibars or 29.92 " of mercury. Used by commercial aircraft above certain altitudes for correct vertical separation of air traffic.

G or G force A measure of acceleration. We all experience 1G (one times the force of gravity) all the time. It is G that 'sticks' people to the 'wall of death' in a fairground and why water does not spill when swung around in a bucket on a rope. G measurements are arithmetical, at 2G your apparent weight doubles, at 5G at 70 kilo person would weigh 350 kilos and be unable to walk. Excessive G can cause the blood to drain from the brain to the lower body causing blackout.

Hunting An aviation term to describe the backward and forward movement of the throttles or thrust lever under autopilot control, attempting to maintain the aircraft at a constant speed.

Jet upset When control of a jet aircraft is lost. Due to the design aerodynamic efficiency of modern jets they accelerate extremely quickly if not properly controlled. At high altitudes they can also quickly bank and enter a dive. Autopilots and vigilant cockpit crew normally prevent this occurrence.

Knot A unit of speed used by ships and aircraft. One knot is one nautical mile (6076 feet) per hour, slightly faster than one statute mile (5280 feet) per hour.

Mach Number	The speed of an aircraft relative to the local speed of sound. Mach .85 indicates the aircraft is flying at 85% of the local speed of sound. Used mostly to express the speed at higher altitudes and for the aircraft's limits and maximum performance.
Mayday	International distress call derived from the French 'm'aidez' – help me.
Minimum Safe Altitude (M.S.A.)	Heights calculated to clear all high ground. This height is 'padded' to allow for barometric variation and for variations due to wind effect over mountains.
NOTAMS	Notices to Airmen provided at flight planning updating which update information on the route and destination.
Position Line	A bearing from a radio beacon or a geographical fix. Drawn on a chart the aircraft's position will lie on this line. When combined with another position line will provide the exact position – a 'fix'.
Round down	The stern end of the flight deck on an aircraft carrier so called because it is bull nosed or round.
Rudder	Situated on the rear of the fin or vertical stabiliser use to offset yaw due to engine failure and to balance turns in piston engine aircraft. Operated by rudder pedals in the cockpit.
Safety Height	A generic term for the minimum height at which it is safe to fly due to the presence of high ground usually increased by factor for safety and to allow for barometric variations over high ground.
SEO	Senior Engineer Officer.
Simulator	A highly sophisticated replica of the aircraft cockpit mounted on hydraulic jacks that simulate aircraft movement. Procedures and emergencies can be simulated and practised at low cost and in safety.
Spool up	A term used to describe the jet engine accelerating. The spools (turbines and compressors) rotating faster and providing greater power as the trust levers are advanced.
Stagger	Throttles not aligned or out of trim.
St Elmo's Fire	A display of static electricity usually visible in cloud on the windscreen as small lightning like flashes. Can take many different forms of display including a bright coloured glow around parts of the aircraft structure.
Tailplane	Also known as horizontal stabiliser. The smaller winglike horizontal surface at the rear of the aircraft. Provides horizontal stability.
Thrust levers	The aeronautical (American) term for throttles.
Transponder	A radar transmitter/receiver required to be fitted to all commercial passenger aircraft. When 'interrogated' by the ground radar it signals a discrete 'blip' on the radar screen for identification purposes. Can also transmit the aircraft's callsign and height. Codes selected by the pilots will give differing 'paints' on the ground controller's radar screen. Code 7700 is the Mayday code.
Trim	The act of 'trimming' the controls so that hand or autopilot input is not required. A properly trimmed aircraft will maintain height and heading without pilot input.
Turb Mode	An autopilot mode which releases the altitude hold and maintains attitude and heading only – gives a smoother ride through turbulence and prevents excessive thrust lever movement.
VOR	Very High Frequency Omnidirectional radio beacon usually also provides distance information from the beacon.
V_1	The takeoff speed at which the aircraft can stop or continue. Past this speed the aircraft is committed to takeoff.
V_r	The correct speed at which to rotate the aircraft for flight.
V_2	The safe climb out speed after takeoff.
V_{ne}	The 'never exceed' speed of the aircraft, it's structural limiting speed.
Weather radar	An aircraft radar in the centimetric band specially designed to detect areas of possible turbulence. It detects areas of water droplets and cloud. Larger water drops in thunderstorms (areas of extreme turbulence) give a stronger return. Can be used for mapping and will display coastlines etc.

THE AUTHOR

On retirement from aviation in 1995 I had spent a total of 41 years in the flying game. The first eight years were spent in the Royal Navy commencing with flying training in the United States at Pensacola, Florida with advanced jet training at Kingsville, Texas. Returning to the UK I spent the next six and a half years operating from a variety of Naval Air Stations with two frontline tours in day fighters operating from the 'light fleet' aircraft carriers, HMS *Bulwark* and HMS *Centaur*. It was during my first tour of duty in 801 Seahawk squadron on Board HMS *Bulwark* that I experienced my one and only aviation catastrophe of the type related in the chapters that follow. This incident is worthy of mention since, in many ways, the circumstances leading up to it and, a subsequent similar accident to the squadron commanding officer, are atypical of many aviation disasters. I have taken the liberty of including the story in the book.

After leaving the Royal Navy in 1962 I spent a short time in journalism and advertising before returning to flying. A short stint operating naval night fighters under contract at Royal Naval Air Station Yeovilton was followed, in 1964, by a 28-year career in Qantas Airways first flying the Boeing 707 and later the Boeing 747. In the later years I was promoted to Check & Training Captain responsible for promotional training of junior pilots to First Officer (co-pilot) and of First Officers to Captain. The duties also included performing the pre-promotion checks on these pilots to see that they had not only the skills, but also the right mental attitude to ensure total safety of their subsequent operations. This awesome responsibility was simply solved in my mind, as well as many of my colleagues, by the simple self question "Would I put my wife and children on an aircraft flown by this person?"

Carrying out First Officer training and training to command was the most fulfilling and enjoyable flying I ever undertook. These pilots, already highly knowledgeable, studied assiduously for their promotional training and spent long hours in the very complex simulators honing their skills and practising every conceivable emergency that could arise. It was rare that any of them could be faulted on their knowledge of the various operations manuals or the required company procedures.

Our job in this area was to ensure that there were no gaps in their knowledge and, if there were, to highlight them. It was in other areas that I had to draw heavily on skills learnt many years before at Royal Air Force Little Rissington where I underwent the Qualified Flying Instructors Course in 1959, and many other skills besides. It was not infrequent that a 'student' would have a temporary difficulty in one area or another but worse, couldn't see the solution to the problem which you were offering, or at least, couldn't get it into his brain. This was often a great challenge which required going 'outside the books'.

The most common example of this was that pilots put themselves into what one might call 'airliner mode'. They flew mostly in a radar environment or under direct control of the various airport controllers and frequently using the autopilot for most of the flight. As a consequence they had abandoned or forgotten many of the basic aspects of airmanship which, as many of the chapters reveal, are often an essential ingredient in resolving a severe crisis in the air and are still essential for routine operations. The not too infrequent 'near misses' and thankfully, far less frequent midair collisions, emphasise that a good 'lookout', especially when flying in the vicinity of airports, is still a vital component of safety when conducting a scheduled airline flight. I had one student who simply would not look out and persisted in flying with his head 'inside the cockpit'.

When I raised this point he explained that he was required to fly to great accuracy and couldn't do this as well if he was always taking his eyes off the instruments. My answer to that was that he had just confessed to not being able to fly any aircraft properly since, a well trimmed aircraft (basic airmanship) will hardly deviate from its height or course if momentarily left to its own devices – especially true of the wonderfully stable aircraft built by the Boeing company. Whilst he was convinced, especially after a demonstration of a well trimmed Boeing 747 flying 'hands off' (but very close to the controls) down an approach path, he still did not look out to my satisfaction. His next sally was that 'We were in a radar environment' intimating that our friends on the ground would look after his aircraft and skin! There had just been a fatal midair collision near Los Angeles when a Boeing 727 had collided with a light aircraft with obvious fatalities, this in a radar environment. I pointed this historical fact out indicating that even under radar collisions can occur. His rejoinder was that the light aircraft pilot had had a heart attack. I commented that I was certain he did – when he looked up and saw his windscreen full of Boeing 727! I was still not getting through and had to devise some way to make this would be Captain a safer pilot.

The opportunity presented itself on a training flight into Singapore. My only regret was that I was unable to give advance warning to the other crewmembers. We were being 'radar vectored' by approach control on a fine clear night. My protégé was doing a good job, but with his eyes continuously inside the cockpit. Without warning I mustered a terrified shout of "**Look out**". My theatrics were obviously very good since his head came up went round like a swivel as he searched the sky for the reason for my call.

"Where, what?" he asked, calling for an indication of the direction of the threat.

"Nowhere, nothing" I replied resuming normal conversational tones, "Just look out."

I had achieved the desired result; the necessity for a good airmanlike lookout was well and truly instilled in his brain, he had thought he was about to die. The other crewmembers, whose eyeballs had come out on stalks, received several cold ales from me after the flight, together with my apologies. I am happy to say this pilot passed his command checks and flew safely for many years with Qantas.

The various 'Emergency Check Lists' and abnormal procedures spelled out in the aircraft operations manuals and carried in a separate booklet ready to hand in the cockpit, deal with almost every crisis that can occur during a flight and will successfully resolve any difficulties. The problems requiring immediate attention are all memorised by the pilots, the less urgent items, to ensure 100% accuracy, are read from the checklist. As the incidents in the chapters vividly illustrate, there are occurrences, fortunately very rare, when something happens which is not catered for in these checklists. The first aircraft to run into severe volcanic ash which the most dramatic results had no procedures laid down to resolve the problem. After that incident, effective procedures were devised and published for each aircraft. It does not pay to be the 'leader of the push' in the aviation game! Thus, each time a major incident or mechanical failure occurs, new and effective safeguards are put in place. Flying becomes safer by the day but that does not mean that new problems will not arise with possibly catastrophic consequences. I saw it as my job as an instructor of airline pilots to prepare my pupils for the unexpected.

During one of many 'briefings' whilst training I would casually ask,

"What is the worst possible thing that could happen to you after you have checked out?"

They would most often reply with what they regarded as the most serious emergency in the checklists. I did not accept that since the procedures were there to deal with that problem. They would search on but find that they couldn't give me an answer that I would accept so I would put a scenario to them.

"Suppose on takeoff from Sydney airport during a maximum weight takeoff, after V1 (go no-go speed), you fly into a large flock of birds and immediately lose two engines?"

Of course the answer is that you are most likely going to ditch in the sea off the end of the runway, but perhaps not. In discussing how to handle this extremely serious emergency with little time available to make the correct decisions, many interesting aspects would come to light. All was not lost. Trading height for speed one could actually get in ground effect which assisted the aircraft's lift. One could bleed the flaps in slowly to reduce drag; they didn't have to be retracted in one 'lump' as the lever was calibrated. Even if the engines had shut down, an instant relight, even with a damaged engine giving some extra thrust was more desirable than 'wet boots' and so it went. Discussing a variety of scenarios prepared the pilot for that 'once in a lifetime' moment when everything went wrong and there were no prepared answers. I was often berated by my superiors for concocting these scenarios, which I regarded, and still do, as the most important part of the training that I was personally giving.

I have no doubt the aircrew who feature in the actual accounts of these airline catastrophes, and who, with one sad exception, brought them to a very successful conclusion, had all prepared themselves for the unexpected and as a result saved their own lives and those of their valued passengers.

A flying club to which I belonged in the 1960's placed a little plaque on the instrument panel of all their aircraft. It read "All aircraft bite fools". Nothing was ever more true. They might have put another plaque alongside it saying "Aircraft don't bite those who are prepared". It was a great pleasure to 'prepare' many young men and women for one of the most interesting and challenging jobs in the world and I believe it made me a better pilot. As the song goes in the musical The King & I, 'By your pupils you are taught!'

Now retired, I play as much golf as I can get away with and annoy my wife by writing books!

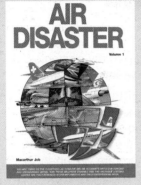
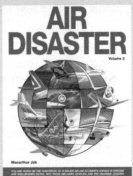
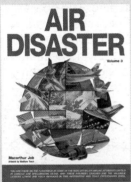
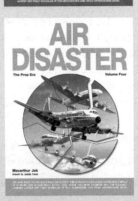
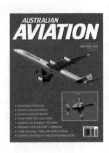